Peng

Cosmetic Surg

COSMETIC SURGERY
Facing the Facts

Christopher Margrave

Penguin Books

To Tatts – my funny Valentine

Penguin Books Ltd, Harmondsworth, Middlesex, England
Viking Penguin Inc., 40 West 23rd Street, New York, New York 10010, U.S.A.
Penguin Books Australia Ltd, Ringwood, Victoria, Australia
Penguin Books Canada Ltd, 2801 John Street, Markham, Ontario, Canada L3R 1B4
Penguin Books (N.Z.) Ltd, 182–190 Wairau Road, Auckland 10, New Zealand

First published 1985

Made and printed in Great Britain by
Cox and Wyman Ltd, Reading
Filmset in Monophoto Photina by
Northumberland Press Ltd, Gateshead,
Tyne and Wear

Contents

Preface

Few surgeons can end a consultation in a clinic or hospital in the certain knowledge that their patients have fully understood the outcome and risks of a particular operation.

The fault lies with both parties. A consultant does not always have enough time to discuss all the implications of a treatment, and even if he does, may find it difficult to explain clearly the nature of a complex problem requiring complicated surgery. Sometimes, if the complaint is a common one and the treatment short and simple, he can soon tire of repetition and lose patience. To make matters worse, the patient, as well as quite often being ill-informed about surgery in general, frequently knows little about cosmetic surgery in particular, which is often portrayed in popular articles and radio and television programmes as either disastrous or nigh miraculous, with the cosmetic surgeon presented as an unscrupulous ogre or a gifted magician. It is not therefore surprising that any interview is liable to end in frustration and confusion.

Surgeons can improve their consultative practice and attitude only by becoming aware of their faults and by submitting themselves to clinical audit systems; patients, on the other hand, can be helped by easily available literature explaining the realities of cosmetic surgery and describing a few common plastic-surgical procedures. All patients should know why they are seeing a surgical specialist, what any treatment might entail, how long they might be absent from home or work and what the complications might be. It is important to know the facts in any treatment of disease that lengthens or saves lives, and mandatory for the patient to be properly informed if faced with the prospect of cosmetic surgery, which may enhance the quality of life but which cannot possibly be considered essential.

This book has been written in an effort to disperse the melodrama and

Preface

mystique, to clarify the truths, expectations and limitations of cosmetic surgery so that hopes may be more realistically fulfilled, and to satisfy the curiosity of the curious.

GENERAL INTRODUCTION

[1]

The History and Language of
Cosmetic Surgery

The cosmetic surgeon is a peculiar and highly specialized animal. Only by studying how he has evolved from other specialists can the patient begin to understand the nature of cosmetic surgery.

In the beginning surgery was surgery: the early surgeons were men who cut and hewed flesh and bone and whose pattern and range of work was limited by the resilience of their patients, who tended to survive in spite of, rather than because of, their operations. It was only as a result of the scientific and biological revolutions of the nineteenth century, and, in particular, the introduction of controlled anaesthesia, that a new era of surgical technology opened. By the middle of the twentieth century no one type of surgeon, apart from the occasional individual of recent memory claiming accomplishment in the surgery of all systems in all seasons, could safely perform every operation, although in countries where medical and surgical services remain poorly developed it was, and still remains, reasonable for a single doctor to offer a necessarily wide range of operations to people who might otherwise suffer or even perish. In countries blessed with greater resources further progress was made through specialization, and it was in this way that the major disciplines of cardiothoracic surgery, ear, nose and throat surgery, orthopaedics, ophthalmology, obstetrics and gynaecology, neurosurgery, dental and oral surgery, and plastic surgery evolved, while general surgery, the original parent, became increasingly restricted to intra-abdominal structures.

The current tendency is to produce sub-specialists and super-specialists who may throw up the occasional technical and therapeutic advance but who run the risk of becoming technically isolated, even stranded, when confronted with a problem that spills beyond the confines of their particular sub-speciality. A great advantage of this trend, however, is in the management of a patient with multiple and complex problems whereby use is made of a team offering wide-ranging specialist expertise, decisions being taken by the team leader to the patient's benefit. But one has to admit that there is a real danger in super-specialization if the implication is committee management of a relatively simple diagnosis, with conflicting advice given to an increasingly confused patient.

To examine the sub-speciality of cosmetic surgery in particular, let us now follow in greater detail the history and evolution of plastic surgery, from which most cosmetic surgeons have sprung.

There are several very early reports of surgical procedures that might come under the heading of plastic surgery. Around 600 BC, in India, Susruta described sixteen different methods of repairing the earlobes of women that had split as a consequence of wearing heavy ear-rings. Hippocrates, in the early fourth century BC, expressed concern about the appearance of abnormal scarring and suggested ways in which this might be improved, and Galen (AD 130–200) wrote extensively on surgical and medical matters including the revision of scars and the correction of eyelid and hand deformities, work that he failed to mention derived from the earlier studies of the Roman medical encyclopaedist Aulus Cornelius Celsus (25 BC–AD 50). In Alexandria, Paul of Aegina (AD 625–90) described how to remove enlarged breast tissue in males, an operation, common today, that can have been performed by him only on cosmetic grounds, while during the Chinese T'ang dynasty of 618–901, Fang Kan acquired a reputation for repairing congenital cleft-lip deformities. However, it is a sad and unpalatable fact that many major advances in reconstructive surgery have taken place through the ingenuity of military surgeons in wartime over the last 400 years, and it is on the shoulders of some of these giants that modern plastic surgeons stand.

Ambroise Paré (1517–90) described new methods of cleaning contaminated war wounds and classified burn injuries according to depth. Sensitive to the hideous facial and limb mutilations among French soldiers, yet aware of his own reconstructive limitations, he designed a large variety of facial and hand prostheses that could at least help the victims to avoid leading a reclusive life. At the same time, in Italy, Gasparo Tagliacozzi rejected the use of nasal prostheses in particular and devised a technique to reconstruct the nose by means of a flap of tissue raised from the patient's upper arm. He too was well aware of the benefit of facial reconstruction and, in his apologia of 1597, *De Curtorum Chirurgia per Insitionem*, wrote: 'We restore, repair and make whole those parts of the face which nature has given, but fortune has taken away, not so much that they may delight the eye but that they may buoy up the spirit and help the mind of the afflicted.' Tagliacozzi was abused and satirized by less enlightened colleagues, while contemporary ecclesiastics accused him of meddling with the destiny of man and the handiwork of God. After his death the published work of Tagliacozzi continued to arouse such animosity among the clergy that his remains were ordered to be exhumed from their convent burial site and reburied in unconsecrated ground. Reconstructive surgery fell into disrepute in Europe, and in 1788 the Paris Faculty of Medicine even banned the teaching and practice of facial surgery.

Further development of surgery designed to reconstruct the maimed was delayed until the Napoleonic Wars, the Austro–Hungarian conflict, the Crimea Campaign and the American Civil War, which produced surgeons concerned not just with increasing the chance of survival for the injured, but improving the quality of the survivors' lives. Among the legendary figures are Carpue and Liston in England; Dieffenbach, von Graefe and Langenbeck in Germany; Dupuytren, Larrey and Marjolin in France; and Mettauer, Buck and Gunning in North America. By the mid nineteenth century Balassa and Lawson had initiated general anaesthesia of a standard high enough to make possible a dazzling variety of reconstructive procedures. However, it was only during and after the First World War that this style of surgery, improved and embellished, received universal recognition as a special surgical art under the heading of plastic and reconstructive surgery. This was the true, unadulterated plastic surgery stemming from the Greek verb 'to mould', and implying the restoration of form destroyed by disease or trauma. The Society of Plastic and Reconstructive Surgery, the first of its kind, was formed in the USA soon after the end of the Great War, and was followed by the formation of similar surgical societies in Britain and Europe. Today there are few countries outside the Third World that do not have their own national societies of plastic surgery.

Many of the early plastic surgeons realized that the surgical methods at their disposal to help in the rehabilitation of young men from the horrors of trench warfare could also be put to good use in civilian life, in the correction of deformities left in the wake of the treatment of degenerative and malignant disease, and in congenital deformities and the unacceptable results of non-pathological phenomena such as ageing and pregnancy. As the range of plastic surgery developed so sub-specialities were inevitably spawned. By the Second World War plastic surgery had become an established and respected speciality, and from then on continued to gather momentum, propagating groups of surgeons with a special interest in either an anatomical area, a particular surgical technique or the treatment of certain types of injury, each group having a sub-speciality name according to the subject. Thus, today, hand surgeons obviously treat problems of this particular area (the dominant parent of this group is orthopaedic rather than plastic), while cranio-facial surgeons treat major deformities of the skull and facial skeleton. Microsurgeons are not diminutive surgical dwarfs, but surgeons who have developed fine reconstructive techniques that can be executed only under magnification, using the operating microscope. Burn surgeons treat burn injuries; head and neck surgeons treat the victims of a cancer in that region.

The final group to acquire independent recognition has been that of cosmetic surgeons, specialists who treat physically fit patients who wish to remedy the effects of ageing or pregnancy, or patients wishing to achieve an appearance that matches their own concept of what is normal or desirable. The goal of cosmetic surgery can be summarized in a plagiarized version of Tagliacozzi's dictum: 'To improve on what nature has given in order to delight the eye, buoy up the spirit and help the mind of the afflicted.' However, in practice, the margin between plastic and cosmetic surgery is ill defined in that the cosmetic surgeon also attempts to improve on certain marks fortune has added to nature, for example in the revision of scars following accidents and minor burns or in the excision of tattoos.

The early cosmetic-surgical practitioners were not always held in great esteem by their colleagues, who accused them of prostituting their skills. In 1900 the celebrated European ear, nose and throat surgeon Dr Joseph reported the results of nasal reduction surgery in ten patients and was greeted with such outrage within his profession that he was compelled to resign from his university post. Even today there are certain cosmetic surgeons who do their sub-speciality a disservice by associating themselves with clinics that advertise in magazines, newspapers and public hoardings and by flaunting an extravagantly flamboyant personal lifestyle. Fortunately, this type is in the minority. The majority lead a life which does not attract the sort of undesirable public and journalistic attention that can rouse justifiable professional jealousy and distaste. They take their sub-speciality as seriously as any other type of surgeon and strive to improve the lot of patients under their care by constant self-criticism and by scientific reappraisal and refinement of their surgical methods.

Some cosmetic surgeons like to call themselves 'aesthetic' surgeons –

a somewhat misleading and pretentious title and one to which no surgical speciality has an exclusive right. By definition, the word 'aesthetic' implies appreciation and criticism of a quality or combination of qualities that afford the keenest delight to the senses. Surgery can be aesthetically appealing according to how skilfully it is executed, how effectively the disease or deformity is treated or corrected, how efficiently a particular function is restored, or, in the most obvious aesthetic connotation, how beautifully a facial feature is remodelled. By these criteria, any operation successfully carried out gives the operator the right to be described as an aesthetic surgeon: but no eye surgeon calls himself an aesthetic ophthalmic surgeon, nor is such a title applied to the many other surgical specialists who might equally well deserve it. Far better that the word 'aesthetic' should be applied to the surgical act in the same way as 'skilful', 'clumsy', 'adept', 'brutal' or any other adjective. However, regardless of the controversy, patients should be aware that aesthetic surgery is now synonymous with cosmetic surgery.

In America, Japan and Australia it is not uncommon for surgeons to proclaim on their professional paper or visiting card not only their main surgical speciality but also their sub-speciality interests. This amounts to a subtle form of advertising by an accepted and perfectly legal system. A visiting card may announce:

George J. Exheimer FACS
Plastic, Cosmetic and Hand Surgery

This leaves the patient, his family and friends in little doubt as to what Dr Exheimer likes to do. In fact surgical territorial and boundary disputes are not a great problem unless it is acknowledged that a surgeon is not qualified to occupy a particular territory. Plastic surgeons have no grounds to resent other specialities overlapping on common sub-speciality interests. After all, plastic surgery is a relatively recent discipline derived from the older schools of ophthalmic, ear, nose and throat, and general surgery, all of which can fairly claim skills in the cosmetic field. Indeed, certain ear, nose and throat surgeons take a special interest in cosmetic surgery of the nose and ears; a few ophthalmic surgeons are expert in the treatment of sagging, unattractively creased ageing eyelids; some maxillo-facial and oral surgeons excel in restructuring the facial skeleton to produce an aesthetically attractive face; the occasional general surgeon restores breast form.

But the main concern of the patient is not necessarily so much that of his surgeon's pedigree, as that he should be completely trained in cosmetic surgery, do the work well and tackle competently any complications that might arise. However, it is sometimes difficult for a prospective patient to judge whether a cosmetic surgeon is fully competent, for while there are rigorous training programmes, including examinations, in almost all the surgical specialities, the national colleges of surgery have no such system for proving all-round ability in cosmetic surgery. A patient must therefore rely on a surgeon's reputation and the recommendation of their own general practitioner or of other patients, and be guided to an individual whose background could be in ear, nose and throat surgery, ophthalmic, maxillo-facial or plastic surgery but who has also taken a particular interest in one or more facets of cosmetic surgery (for more specific guidelines see Appendix A, 'Routes to Surgery in Britain').

Homo cosmeticus is now identified, albeit in necessarily vague terms. In later chapters other dimensions will be added by describing the tools of his trade, the details of his work and the demands, motivation and behaviour of his patients. Meanwhile it might be of interest and even of some benefit for potential patients to understand the language of cosmetic surgery. A comprehensive Linguaphone course is not necessary, but some key words and phrases could help.

Any patient should be suspicious of a cosmetic surgeon who throws up a smokescreen of jargon, but should also realize that the words can be decoded if the roots and derivations of named operations and procedures are understood. Much current medical terminology stems from Greek and Latin, which have always been associated with science in Europe and were the languages in which all medicine was taught until the great European centres of medical education were established in the seventeenth century, when clinical medicine began to be taught at the patient's bedside in the country's own mother tongue rather than through perfunctory lectures in Latin given in an auditorium. Even in the early part of this century prospective medical students still had to be well grounded in Greek and Latin.

It therefore comes as no surprise that the word 'cosmetic' stems from the Greek verb *kosmein*, to adorn or decorate. *Plassein* is the Greek verb to mould and *plastikos* relates to moulding: by adding '-plasty' to the Greek name for an anatomical component one arrives at the technical term for a plastic or cosmetic operation. *Blepharon* is the Greek for an eyelid: so blepharoplasty is an operation to improve the appearance of eyelids. *Rhis* is Greek for a nose: hence the operation of rhinoplasty. The patient can now begin to understand the meaning of operative terms. Mammoplasty becomes clear once it is known that *mamma* means a breast, even if the term is a compound of Latin and Greek (*mamma* coming from the Latin). Abdominoplasty and vaginoplasty speak for themselves.

Ektome comes from the Greek meaning to excise or cut off; by adding this to the word for the relevant anatomical part a surgeon's intention becomes obvious. Rhinectomy is fortunately a very rare procedure, but lipectomy is a common cosmetic operation in which 'lip-' derives from *lipos*, meaning fat. It is also important to understand from which part of the body the fat is to be removed – from the abdomen (abdominal lipectomy), from the arms (brachial lipectomy) or from under the chin (submental lipectomy). Knowing that *rhytis* means a wrinkle and that the word 'cervical' comes from *cervix*, meaning neck, a patient will be undaunted by the most arrogant and awe-inspiring cosmetic surgeon; for when the latter offers a cervicofacial rhytidectomy and a submental lipectomy, the patient will know at once that some fat will be cut from under the chin and wrinkles removed from the face and neck: in other words, the surgeon will be offering a facelift.

[2]

Motivations and Psychological Aspects

A question that cosmetic surgery certainly raises is why a fit and healthy person whose looks fall well within the range of the normal should ever choose to undergo an inessential operation, with all the discomfort and risks that go with it, when to so many others with much better grounds for complaint the idea is unthinkable. Looking good may help one feel good but this cannot adequately explain the lengths to which people go in order to achieve a transformation, and the true underlying motive remains a mystery to psychiatrists, psychologists and cosmetic surgeons alike. However, psychological and behavioural studies have done much to make the concepts underlying cosmetic surgery easier to understand.

The psychologist explains the motivation for cosmetic surgery according to two main theories. The first overlaps with socio-anthropological ideas and takes account of environmental influences and pressures on a person making a decision to consult a cosmetic surgeon; social, cultural, racial and religious aspects and the context of employment and family are all investigated and where applicable interpreted as motivating factors. Psychiatrists of this attitude can be said to belong to the environmental or sociogenic school.

The other theory is based on the longer-term and more remote influences that may have moulded a patient's character, and requires the psychiatrist to delve more deeply into the past and the unconscious. Members of this psychogenic school respect Freudian analysis and encourage the patient to re-enact infant and childhood life, to remember the attitudes and moods of parents, details of time spent at school and of relationships with childhood friends, before then analysing the circumstances of each stage of early and adult life. The motivation for cosmetic surgery as explained along these lines is sometimes difficult to understand, as the language is often couched in clichéd, negative jargon which may be of help to the psychiatrist in classifying different patterns of behaviour, but which is of limited value to the interested layman and particularly to the surgeon. To be told that a woman has a profound and irredeemable sense of hostility, repression or guilt or has acquired a compulsive obsessional neurosis does not rationalize her motivation for surgery in any easily understood way.

However, no contemporary psychiatrist belongs exclusively to one or the other school but uses information from both in the knowledge that every individual is unique and cannot be conveniently categorized, and that the reason why any person turns to cosmetic surgery is necessarily multidimensional. To take an extreme case, the occasional patient hunting desperately for a cosmetic surgeon will have an abnormal and unreasonable preoccupation with part of his or her anatomy, often the nose, and display behaviour verging on the psychotic (known as dysmorphophobic behaviour). Cosmetic surgery does nothing to help such patients, sometimes even makes matters worse, and the psychiatrist plays an important part in guiding them towards psychotherapy or treatment by drugs, and in distinguishing them from other patients who can genuinely be helped by cosmetic surgery. In the mid 1970s the danger of failing to identify dysmorphophobia was highlighted by a report concerning a highly reputable Spanish cosmetic surgeon who operated in good faith on the nose of a young man who, unknown to him, had powerful latent psychotic tendencies. Although the surgery was uneventful and the planned results achieved, the patient was so dissatisfied that he shot the surgeon dead.

The most plausible explanation for a person's motivation for cosmetic surgery has come, not from a psychiatrist, but from an English plastic surgeon. Basing his ideas on the literature published by psychiatrists interested in this aspect of behaviour and on information gathered from detailed personal interviews with many patients undergoing a wide variety of cosmetic operations, he has described a sequence of events which, depending on the degree of self-consciousness of the patient, ultimately lead to surgery.

First of all one must understand the causes of abnormal appearance, and these can be summed up as follows:

1. Abnormalities evident at birth such as birthmarks or a cleft lip and palate.
2. Abnormalities arising from an accident or that are the direct result of

disease or of treating disease. Examples are the scarring resulting from a traffic accident or a burn, the pock-marks left on the face after severe adolescent acne, or the loss of a breast by mastectomy for breast cancer.

3. Normal and natural phenomena which are an unavoidable part of ageing or motherhood, for example the effect of pregnancy on the shape of the breasts and contour of the abdomen, or that of ageing on the face and body.

4. Developmental disproportion, i.e., the unequal growth of breasts at puberty or the development of enormous breasts that are inappropriate to the build of a young woman.

Most patients can vividly remember the age at which they first became self-conscious about an unwanted physical feature and may recall a number of events that were responsible for their growing self-consciousness. Criticism by others, usually in the form of teasing, plays a large part in this respect and may be friendly with no intention of malice, involving jokes and leg-pulling, or frankly hostile, involving public ridicule and the use of brutal nicknames. Covert criticism in the form of staring or whispered comments behind one's back can be just as harmful. During this time patients become self-critical and compare their appearance with others', often in the hope of meeting someone with a similar or more obvious problem and thereby finding consolation and reassurance that they are not, after all, 'abnormal'. Self-consciousness can also result from a situation where the signal given to others by a patient's appearance bears no relationship to his or her personality. For example, a young woman with unusually large breasts may be mistakenly taken for a 'good-time girl', or a man with puffy, baggy eyelids having a social drink in a bar may be thought a potential, if not a hopeless, alcoholic.

The inappropriate and offensive response in others to an individual's appearance induces a variety of defence mechanisms of which the most common is camouflaging the focus of attention by means of clothes, make-up, and postures and gestures that disguise and distract. The patient may go to extremes and adopt atypical and artificial behaviour as a compensatory defence mechanism – like the small-breasted woman who, having a feeling of diminished femininity, becomes promiscuous; or the young man with an ugly facial birthmark who jokes about it before others find the chance to do so; or the person with facial scars caused by an accident whose manner becomes so aggressive and tough that no one dares to comment. A usual reflex is the restriction of lifestyle and the deliberate avoidance of situations that are known to be embarrassing. Thus a boy who is unmercifully teased at school on account of his prominent ears may play truant; a young man with slightly full breasts (a relatively common occurrence in adolescence) will avoid swimming; a woman with flaccid, stretch-marked breasts and abdomen will often undress only in the dark. However, some activities are unavoidable, and it is on these occasions, when an untoward appearance attracts glances and remarks from strangers, that life can be misery.

The cumulative effect of all this unwanted attention and criticism is to erode the patient's image of self to the point where he or she feels unattractive, unloved, insecure and somehow inferior, and can ultimately result in total loss of self-confidence. This may in turn lead to withdrawal and secrecy: patients will hide their distress and fears even from their closest confidant (including, unfortunately, their doctor, who may be the only person in a position to give proper guidance and help) and may consequently develop difficulties in personal relationships, finding it stressful both to meet new people and to maintain established friendships. Teenagers will often be unable to relate to the opposite sex, while adults may find obstacles to marriage and, more particularly, sexual relationships.

The decision whether or not to undergo cosmetic surgery may also be influenced by one final factor – aesthetic sensibility – which, itself qualified by the aesthetic values of race, culture and society, affects the way in which individuals view themselves and judge their image. A person with heightened sensibility is more likely to feel self-conscious about a defect than one in whom the sense is less acute.

Aesthetic sensibility is a phenomenon peculiar to human beings in their pursuit of objects and experiences that give delight to the senses. Sources of pleasure vary enormously from one individual to another, since background, parental influence and racial and cultural preferences all have a part in shaping a person's aesthetic standards, and these are of course infinite in kind. There can be no unanimity over what constitutes the beautiful: one can only reaffirm that beauty is very much in the eye of the beholder. So wide-ranging are conceptions of beauty that the heavy build of an Egyptian belly-dancer will be a thing of loveliness in Egypt but not in Thailand, where smallness and delicacy are perhaps the most desirable attributes of the female body. Similarly the enormous bulk of a Japanese Sumo wrestler will be greatly admired in Japan but will not compare, in

Western eyes, with the muscle-bound physique of a professional weight-lifter. Such racial variations are significant in the practice of cosmetic surgery, and in France, for example, where small breasts are considered beautiful, breast augmentation is less in demand than in the USA, where big is beautiful. This is borne out by the fact that the average size of a breast implant used by cosmetic surgeons in France is 140 cc as against 260 cc in the USA. However, racial characteristics identifying a particular ethnic group are often modified, for whatever reason, to resemble those of another: Oriental eyelids may be given an Occidental look, a broad, flat nose changed to a narrower, more prominent one, a large nose made smaller.

In our own working lives, youth and good looks are often regarded as important attributes where personal success is concerned; this is a direct result of the influence of advertising on a susceptible consumer who is led to believe that youth + beauty equals energy, and energy + knowledge equals business efficiency. This is less the case in university hierarchies, where hard work, experience and genuine talent are the main yardsticks for higher appointment. But then, functional aesthetic values vary from one community to the next as much as any other aesthetic value. The youth and beauty cult may be misbegotten but it continues to be regarded as an asset in some commercial endeavours, and aspiring or vulnerable employees are often driven into the hands of cosmetic surgeons in an attempt to transform themselves according to the aesthetic standards of employers, clients or public. So important is appearance that in some communities where cosmetic surgery is much in demand, where private enterprise flourishes and where competition is fierce, surgeons themselves inveigle colleagues into changing a feature or two so that prospective patients may not be put off by whatever flaws they may have. There are also those who consult a cosmetic surgeon in the belief that a marriage or close personal relationship will be salvaged if they adjust their looks to satisfy the expressed aesthetic preferences of their partner. In this case surgery does not provide an easy solution, since the problem lies elsewhere.

Whether an individual feels strongly enough actually to take the irreversible step and undergo cosmetic surgery obviously depends on a combination of all the above-mentioned factors, on how acutely he or she feels about the 'abnormality', and on what sort of guidance is given by the doctor. Whatever the case, it must be said that cosmetic surgery is not the prerogative of the rich and famous; the myth of exclusivity is due to the journalist's readiness to report anything that seems in the least sensational in the lives of the rich and famous. Neither is it the obsession of the neurotic and the mentally unstable or a service restricted to consumer-conscious Western democracies: cosmetic surgery is practised in China* and in Russia and its European satellites. In fact cosmetic surgery can no longer be regarded as the frivolous self-indulgence of the privileged few but as a commodity that is socially and psychologically justifiable and that is in some cases a distinct necessity.

*On a recent journey to Shanghai the author was shown a suite of private rooms at the top of a new hospital block which was available for state-subsidized and fee-paying patients undergoing cosmetic surgery.

[3]

The Ageing of Skin

The search for increased longevity and eternal youth has preoccupied the human race possibly since the day it became aware of the impact and inevitability of old age, but despite the great advances of the last century in the understanding, prevention and treatment of disease there are still no pills, potions, unguents or prayers to halt or reverse its progress, nor are there any explanations for the mechanism of ageing – a progressive process that eventually kills us all.

Do we inherit genes that dictate our lifespan? Are there natural biological errors in the synthesis of proteins? Do somatic mutations noted by Darwin as an expression of gradual gross evolutionary change occur more frequently at the cellular level than might be appreciated? Do hormones or built-in immunological patterns control our destiny, or is it simply that waste products accumulate in dividing cells, slowing them down and eventually extinguishing their lives as components of heart, lung, artery and muscle? All these are hypotheses that have yet to be proved or disproved by gerontologists, but, whatever the theories of ageing in general, no one dies of old skin, and it is remarkable how rapidly the cells of the epidermis (the outermost layer of the skin) continue to be shed and replaced, albeit at a slower rate, in late old age itself.

The manifestations of ageing skin are not a consequence of epidermal function but of changes in the deeper layer called the dermis, which is of variable thickness in man but of such thickness and strength in larger animals that it can be made into leather for hard-wearing items such as shoes, sandals, belts and straps. The ruggedness of the dermal component of skin is due to a convoluted, coiled network of collagen fibres which forms 80 per cent of its bulk and which, in combination with interspersed and finer elastic fibres, allows the skin to stretch and relax. Free movement of the system is ensured by the lubricating action of a surrounding interstitial fluid known as ground substance. The meshwork of collagen and elastic fibres in a young person lengthens and expands in stretching and bending movements but returns to its original dimensions on relaxation much as a new woollen sweater regains its shape. However, with age, the collagen fibres lose their coils at rest* and the accompanying elastic fibres their elasticity, so that the dermis and skin as a whole gradually become less able to snap back into shape after stretching, growing ever more slack and wrinkled. This effect is compounded by the reduction in volume and quality of the oil-like ground substance and also by the increasing inefficiency of the collagen-producing cells, which causes the dermal layer to become progressively thinner. The process can be likened to that whereby the fibres of the sweater, now well worn and repeatedly washed, become attenuated and fixed in their elongated state at the areas of greatest movement, and particularly at the elbows. (While the worn-out garment can finally be discarded and replaced, this is not unfortunately possible with old, tired skin, and its owner must either learn to live with it or have the unacceptably baggy bits cut out by a cosmetic surgeon, in the understanding that the remaining skin is just as old and will eventually slacken and crease again.)

The net result of this physico-chemical change within the dermis is that the skin develops fixed laxity rather than reversible extensibility, and wrinkled, deep creases are formed in areas of greatest mobility such as the forehead, face, neck, knees and elbows. The only consolation that can be gleaned from this process is that the diminished elasticity and tone of old dermis make for a finer and more aesthetic scar after accidental injury or deliberate surgical incision than is possible in a young person, in whom the more active collagen and elastic fibres tend to stretch and distort the weakened points of the scar to larger and uglier dimensions.

Complicating the issue is the centripetal redistribution, with time, of body fat, which is lost earlier and to a greater degree from the limbs, face

---

*The fundamental chemical change in ageing collagen which contributes to its physical alteration is the phenomenon known as 'cross-linkage', whereby its molecules become more rigidly bonded to each other. Molecular cross-linkage is abnormal in many forms of disease as well as occurring naturally in health, and is a fascinating but ill-understood process that has been identified as one of the many theoretical causes of ageing. In that collagen makes up a ubiquitous biological framework, particularly in joints and the walls of arteries and veins, the secret of longer life may lie with the control of cross-linkage and of the cells which manufacture this substance.

and extremities while being deposited more readily in the region of the abdomen and trunk, and whose changes not only contribute to the characteristic body shape associated with old age but also leave in their wake redundant folds of skin that are more apparent at an earlier age in women than in men. This natural centripetalism is added to by the effects of gravity, such that the soft tissues of the face, trunk and buttocks shift downwards in inexorable if almost imperceptible fashion, rather like a greatly decelerated lava flow. The skin is adversely affected by all these changes: the movement of fat from the face to the neck exaggerates the wrinkles and creases of the cheeks and jowls, while the skin of the upper arms and thighs is unable to take up the slack after loss of its underlying fatty support and in extreme cases may hang in flapping folds.

In women of childbearing age the ageing process can be speeded up in the region of the abdomen and breasts by the effects of pregnancy and breastfeeding: abdominal skin distended by pregnancy does not always return to its former tautness and frequently hangs in stretch-marked folds that cannot be improved by the most rigorous diet or exercise, while previously full, well-formed breasts can shrink to mere flaps after breastfeeding.

Other structures in the skin are also susceptible to ageing. The cells that lie in the sweat glands become less active after the menopause and after the age of fifty in men, imparting a drier texture to the skin. Surprisingly, the cells of the sebaceous glands responsible for keeping the hair follicles oiled remain efficient well into old age, although as is well known the quality of the hair itself and the pattern of hair growth change dramatically with age.

The colour and distribution of scalp hair is determined by genes: the chances are that a prematurely greying or balding scalp in a young man (receding hair at the temples is often found in twenty-year-olds) will already have been noted in older relatives. Hormones also influence hair growth, as demonstrated by the fact that male-pattern baldness does not occur in eunuchs and that baldness fails to progress after castration in adult life. Greying is caused by progressive loss of pigment cells, or melanocytes, from the hair bulb and occurs in 50 per cent of men and women by the age of fifty, with half the hair affected. Balding is equally common in men, and over half the male population has obvious baldness at the front and sides of the scalp by the same age. Women bald to a lesser degree, but 60 per cent between the ages of forty and seventy have detectable recession at the temples. Armpit, body and pubic hair reaches its peak in density and volume by the age of forty and then gradually thins out, particularly in the region of the trunk. After sixty 33 per cent of women lose all armpit hair as against 5 per cent of men, but compensate in 40 per cent of cases by developing coarse facial hair. Meanwhile the only hair to proliferate in older men is that in the ears, eyebrows and nose.

With time the pigment cells of the skin begin to behave unpredictably, leaving an uneven patchy pigmentation, particularly over exposed areas such as the hands and face. More important, they also decrease in number at the rate of 10 per cent every ten years from the age of thirty, with important consequences. One of the responsibilities of these cells is to protect the skin from the harmful effects of sunlight, which is why a dark skin is so useful in equatorial and semi-equatorial regions. As the population of pigment cells diminishes, so the skin becomes increasingly susceptible to damage by sunlight and to cancer in the form of tumours, a disadvantage hardly offset by the fact that the loss of pigment cells also leads to the number of raised brown moles being gradually reduced to an average of four per person over the age of fifty. (Moles are very rarely seen in people over eighty.)

Benign skin lesions proliferate with age, and every adult over the age of sixty-five can expect to develop one or more growths, whether skin tags, raised red spots, greasy brown spreading patches, flat dark areas like an ink-blot or dry, flaking, black verrucous marks. More worrying is the growing incidence of malignant or cancerous lesions, particularly in old age, not unconnected with excessive exposure to sunlight.

Although nothing has been proven to halt or slow down the ageing of skin, one factor is universally acknowledged to hasten its effects, namely sunlight. (The damaging component, ultraviolet radiation, is incidentally also emitted by the light sources of some of the increasingly popular sunbeds, and anyone using such devices to maintain an all-season tan may be accelerating the ageing process to exactly the same degree as a regular sun-worshipper.) The deleterious effects of sunbathing start to become obvious in middle age, with wrinkles appearing in repeatedly exposed areas well in advance of those in areas normally protected from the sun, such as the buttocks. Of more serious import, however, is the greatly increased risk of skin cancer in Caucasians living in countries near the equator who regularly expose themselves to the sun; and in South Africa, Australia and the southern states of the USA the various types of skin cancer have become worryingly frequent in white skins. All this is common knowledge to any doctor, and one now long-retired plastic surgeon in Britain believed the danger to be so great that he actually carried out a one-man crusade during his holidays and summer weekends, parading beaches and open-air swimming pools exhorting sunbathers to cover up. Recently, in certain Australian states, government-sponsored campaigns similar to those initiated in Britain against smoking or drinking and driving have been set up to alert the public both to the long-term hazards of prolonged exposure to the sun and to the early detection of skin cancer. Other countries have now begun to follow Australia's example.

The adage that no one dies of old skin should therefore be qualified to read that no one dies of under-exposed old skin, and today's young owners of beautifully bronzed skin should realize that they will be the prematurely wrinkled and cancer-prone individuals of tomorrow.

[4]

Tools of the Trade

One of the questions most likely to exasperate a cosmetic surgeon is sometimes asked by a patient after a lengthy consultation explaining the site and characteristics of the scars to be expected after a particular operation: 'But surely I'm not going to have any scars? After all, I'm having plastic surgery, aren't I?'

It is not the fault of the patient that such a question should be asked but rather of the mystic aura that plastic surgeons have somehow acquired through the more sensational publicity surrounding their work. They are not magicians with magic wands: they are surgeons who remodel flesh and use instruments identical to those of any other type of surgeon, and·who in so doing destroy cells and tissues which repair themselves extraordinarily efficiently but which are inevitably left permanently scarred (see Chapters 6 and 7, 'Scars' and 'Skin Grafts'). Hopefully, in learning something about the style and action of the tools used in surgery, patients may begin to realize that there is no mystery, and that a cut made by a plastic surgeon heals with a scar in exactly the same way as a cut made by any other surgeon.

The Scalpel Blade

Many instruments of varied complexity and cost are available for the purposes of surgical incision and dissection, but the favourite tool for these is simply a sharp scalpel blade, which as a hand-held instrument has a pleasing precision and accuracy unmatched even by recent innovations such as the computer-controlled laser. Similarly a sculptor has access to a whole range of power-driven instruments with which to carve and shape a block of stone or marble, but the tools for which he will most commonly reach are the familiar hammer and chisel. No two sculptures produced by the carver will be identical: nor can two operations ever be the same by virtue of the biological multiformity of the human species and the infinite variation in the pattern of disease. For this reason, individually planned surgery accurately executed with the help of simple and easily handled instruments is the goal, and until a cutting device is introduced which leaves no trace or scar in human tissue the scalpel blade will remain the surgeon's favourite tool.

The Skin-graft Knife

Until thirty or forty years ago skin grafts were taken with the aid of long blades fitted with a handle. There are still surgeons who prefer to harvest skin by this elementary means and who yet manage to cut grafts with greater accuracy and skill than some younger surgeons using powered dermatomes, but the most popular type of skin-graft knife today is one with a guard and a roller guide that can be set at variable distances from the knife edge to allow grafts of any thickness to be cut. The principle is similar to that of the old-fashioned butcher's bacon-slicer or of the continental cheese knife used to cut wafer-thin slices of soft cheese.

Other dermatomes (skin-cutting apparatus) have been produced in an effort to make the process quick, easy and foolproof, and include the drum dermatome and the air-powered or electrically driven dermatome. These powered machines are a little like the electric clippers used by hairdressers to trim the hairs on the back and sides of the neck and are quite useful in cases where a large number of skin grafts are required, for example in resurfacing an area following an extensive burn. However, it is surprising how many surgeons return to the guarded knife where only a small skin graft is needed, as in covering a limited area such as an unhealed skin ulcer or the defect remaining after excision of a large skin tumour.

Air Drills

In spite of the understandable reluctance of surgeons to give way to modern technology in practising the art of surgery, some innovations are regarded as welcome additions to the equipment of the operating theatre. One of these is the high-speed drill, propelled by the release of air through a valve at the head of a cylinder containing compressed air and controlled either at the level of the valve, or by a foot pedal, or through manipulation of a lever close to its end. The whole system is in fact identical to that used by dentists for drilling holes in teeth, down to the fine spray of water intended to cool the tip of the rapidly rotating head. Cosmetic and plastic surgeons find the air drill invaluable in performing procedures such as planing skin or cutting bone to shape, and attachments are available for each purpose. For example, a rotating cylinder or small sphere coated in metallic or diamond particles attached to the end of the drill will help remove the surface irregularities of an acne-pitted face and smooth the contours of some scars, and a small saw or cutting drill will enable bones of the face and jaw to be divided along pre-planned lines and, once relocated, immobilized with the help of wires tied through holes drilled in appropriate sites.

Surgical Diathermy

When skin is cut (or any other organ for that matter), blood is released which, if uncontrolled, floods the wound and prevents the surgeon from proceeding further; not only that: if a large vessel is cut, excessive blood loss will endanger the patient. Even after the skin has been closed blood may continue to leak into the wound, where it will collect as a large clot (or haematoma), delay healing of the lesion, threaten the quality of the repair and act both as a source of pain and as a potential focus for infection. Effective arrest of bleeding is therefore essential and can be achieved either by closing the end of the artery or vein with a knotted ligature or by sealing it with a high-frequency electric current passed through the body of the patient between two electrodes. This is not as dangerous as it sounds, for the current is of such frequency that it causes no damage except at the working point of the 'live' electrode (usually a pair of dissecting forceps), where it generates only enough heat to coagulate small bleeding vessels. The current from the live electrode travels through the patient to a large, 'indifferent' electrode in the form of a thin, flexible metallic sheet placed in contact with the thigh or buttock, where its density is so small as to have no warming or otherwise perceptible effect on the skin. A patient under general anaesthesia will not be aware of the presence of the indifferent electrode, but conscious patients undergoing minor plastic surgery using a local anaesthetic will be told of the plate and reassured that there will be no untoward sensation at the moment of diathermy coagulation. The only evidence of its use will be a short buzz as the surgeon completes the circuit with a foot pedal or trigger.

The principle of diathermy can be put to further use by modifying the current so that at the live electrode an arc is struck between its point and the underlying tissues. This arc is so hot that it has the effect of cutting and simultaneously sealing the small points of bleeding. Cutting diathermy is rarely used on the skin as the resulting scars are worse than after incision with a scalpel, but for dividing deeper tissues it is a surgical asset.

Cryosurgery

Extreme cold destroys tissue, as anyone will confirm who has experienced or witnessed frostbite, and, if properly controlled, can be put to clinical use in treating superficial lesions of the skin. Tissue death from cold occurs as a result of cellular damage due to formation of ice crystals, cellular dehydration and eventual rupture of the membrane surrounding the cells, and can be induced by application of liquid air, carbon dioxide snow and liquid nitrogen. Unfortunately, these methods have proved to be a little haphazard in that they can also lead to freezing of the normal structures surrounding the target, resulting in more extensive scarring than is normally desired. A more accurate technique has therefore been developed which uses a range of fine metallic rods with variously shaped tips that can be cooled to the desired temperature and applied to an unwanted skin growth. The duration of contact of the rod, or cryoprobe, is crucial and the operator has to judge from experience how many seconds will be necessary to destroy a particular growth. However there is still an element of 'hit-and-miss' in terms of preserving surrounding normal tissue, and although the cryoprobe remains a useful surgical tool it has been largely superseded by the more precise but infinitely more expensive medical laser.

Lasers

Science fiction and television documentaries have so popularized the laser that the doctor can sympathize with a patient who might believe it to be the ultimate surgical tool. In fact the laser has not realized its full promise and at present has only a limited role to play in surgery.

The laser (the name comes from the original description of the process as Light Amplification by Stimulated Emission of Radiation) is an instrument which transmits an intense beam of pure, non-divergent, coherent monochromatic light waves of the same length, travelling in complete phase and in the same direction. It first appeared in 1960, since when an array of powerful systems has been developed for use in industry, defence and science. Lasers of medical relevance are weaker but are nonetheless sufficiently strong to warrant considerable caution, and the Department of Health and Social Security has issued guidelines and safety precautions, while a new group called the British Medical Laser Association promotes their correct and safe use in the treatment of patients.

Almost all medical lasers use gas as the active medium, which according to its type determines the wavelength of the coherent beam and thereby defines its therapeutic role. Many kinds of laser have been tried and tested but at present only two have found their way into the repertoire of the cosmetic surgeon. The first is the carbon dioxide laser, which generates infra-red light, absorbed rapidly by water, and which destroys tissues by vaporizing cells. The beam seals the cut and can be controlled with the help of an operating microscope to give fine, precise and relatively bloodless results. This type of laser has a place in the excision of large tumours and of deeply damaged skin in burn victims but is no substitute for the old-fashioned surgical scalpel in the cutting of skin. It has also been used to remove unwanted tattoos but, like any other treatment, replaces these with a scar. The second type is the argon laser, which emits a blue-green beam that is selectively absorbed by its complementary colour, red. This property is useful in the treatment of patients with extensive red facial birthmarks (port-wine stains), and works by selective coagulation of the small, abnormal blood vessels contained in them. The results are promising but have not been shown to provide the definitive solution to this difficult problem.

There is a third, very low-powered, type of laser which uses helium, neon and gallium arsenide as the medium to provide what is called a 'cold beam'. The beauty salons and 'cosmetic clinics' which use this laser claim that it rejuvenates the face, but it has no proven effect whatsoever on ageing skin, and all that can be said in its defence is that it does no harm.

All medical lasers are expensive instruments and their purchase is difficult to justify unless they can be shown to have an outstanding advantage over a cheaper, more conventional tool. However, despite this reservation, further research and trial will continue in this field until the perfect surgical cutting instrument is found that leaves no trace of its passage.

Lights and Loupes

A surgeon must always be able to see what he is doing, and for this reason makes use of specially designed operating-theatre illumination and an assistant to retract the surrounding tissues and keep the operative site clear of blood for easy surgical access. Where operations on small structures within small, deep, dark holes are concerned (for example the tiny bones and delicate membranes in the recesses of the middle ear, the province of the ear, nose and throat [ENT] surgeon), conventional lighting is inadequate and a more powerful and more easily directed source, now available in the form of fibre-optic systems, is essential. In such circumstances normal unaided vision is also insufficient for the very fine surgery required and the operator has to boost this with instruments similar to those of the watchmaker, who for generations has used a magnifying eye-glass and microscope as an aid to his work. Some of these have been modified to facilitate even more delicate sections, which has led to the growth of a new surgical sub-speciality called microsurgery. Thus the ENT surgeon is able to add not only flexible fibre-optic illumination to his repertoire of instruments but also operating microscopes and binocular magnifying lenses mounted on a spectacle frame, otherwise known as operating loupes.

Plastic surgeons acknowledge the major surgical advances that have come through fibre-optic illumination, optical magnification and micro-instrumentation and are well versed in microsurgical techniques. The cosmetic surgeon has little use for microsurgery but finds the better lighting, the operating loupes and some of the finer instruments a great bonus. The fibre-optic light, for example, connected via a cable to a power source, can be attached to a headband so as to give brilliant illumination as the surgeon peers into a pocket, or, alternatively, fixed to a retractor so that, when inserted into a cavity of the nose, beneath facial flaps in the course of a facelift or under the breast prior to augmentation, it will allow the area to be visualized more clearly. Similarly, magnifying surgical loupes and selected micro-instruments can be used to advantage in the meticulous surgery required, for example, in eyelid reduction. None of these aids, of course, can substitute for good, basic technique but they can help the surgeon to bridge the difference between a very good result and a perfect one.

Sutures and Clips

In closing a wound after an operation the surgeon has to bear in mind both the strength of the ties necessary to hold the edges together until healing has taken place and the final aesthetic appearance of the scar. Although adhesives have been tried none are yet sufficiently reliable to substitute for the time-honoured and well-tested suture guided into the skin and deeper structures with the help of a sharp, curved needle.

Sutures are classified according to whether they are absorbable, non-absorbable, natural or synthetic, and are available in a wide and constantly expanding range. Not a month goes by without yet another suture or ligature appearing on the market, but surgeons are creatures of habit, and of the natural absorbable sutures used the most common remains catgut (obtained not from stray cats as some animal-lovers believe but from the middle layer of the foregut of government-inspected sheep). Twisted strands of polyglycolic acid are the most frequently used synthetic absorbable suture but are not broken down as rapidly as catgut, which normally disappears after a few weeks, and may persist for several months. This is of some relevance to the patient, for although absorbable sutures are used to reinforce the wound only in its deeper layers they sometimes work their way towards the surface of the skin before natural dissolution and are discharged as tiny, tattered threads, not unreasonably causing concern in the patient. If this happens, the latter can safely be reassured that nothing is seriously amiss. Because of their unpredictable absorption period, these types of sutures are seldom used in the skin.

Before the advent of synthetic non-absorbable surgical materials the surgeon happily used natural sutures of cotton, linen, silk or hair, but even the most conservative individual could not deny the advantages of the new synthetics, and particularly of those derived from the polyolefins as polyethylene and polypropylene. Synthetic non-absorbable sutures pass smoothly and with little friction through tissues, are not only easy to insert but easy to remove and, with the exception of silk, have almost completely replaced the natural non-absorbable type.

At the end of a protracted major cosmetic operation such as an abdominoplasty, breast reduction or facelift, the prospect of closing the long, multiple incisions can be slightly daunting, since every suture must be placed in just the right position and secured and knotted at just the right tension. It was therefore with some relief that cosmetic surgeons welcomed the appearance of surgical clips, which can be rapidly applied in sequence, reducing the time and tedium of conventional suturing. However, clips are sometimes a little painful to remove and, of greater significance, leave unacceptable marks. Thus although they have not been rejected altogether, they are used selectively in places where the scar can be reasonably well concealed, as in the bikini area after an abdominoplasty or in the hair-bearing area of the scalp after a browlift.

Drugs and Dressings

Surgeons are not just technicians, they are also fully trained doctors familiar with the more common diseases and disorders that are treated by non-surgical remedies, and can wield the prescription pad or treatment chart as well as anyone else (though not where rarer or more complex medical problems are concerned, of course, and here a physician's help is requested). Thus a surgeon is well equipped to cope, for example, in the treatment of infection or the relief of pain and anxiety.

One of the surgeon's main responsibilities is to see that the patient recovers quickly and uneventfully from an operation, and that the wounds heal soundly and with as little discomfort as possible: surgical treatment does not end with the knotting of the last suture, and the wound must be kept clean, sterile and insulated with proper dressings until it has healed sufficiently for the sutures to be removed. The best dressings are simple, cheap, widely available, and comfortable to apply and remove, and take the form of a tailored, sterile, non-adherent inner layer overlaid with loosely woven fabric to absorb any leaking fluid and blood and kept in place with sticky tapes or plaster. The three components of the dressing can be applied either in one unit, as in the case of an elastoplast with a central pad within an adhesive surround, or separately, and come in different shapes and sizes suitable for any dimension of wound. If the dressing becomes excessively stained, contaminated or smelly it can be removed with relatively little pain, allowing the wound to be cleaned and re-dressed. Where there is a significant risk of wound infection, the inner non-stick layer can be impregnated with an antibiotic.

There is no scientific or anecdotal evidence to support the belief that certain dressings, medicines, lotions or potions can accelerate the rate of healing of a wound. Only by eliminating local factors that inhibit healing, such as infection, foreign bodies, dead tissue and blood clots, and by improving the general health of the patient can a surgeon provide optimum conditions for a wound to heal at its normal rate.

Silicone Implants

Another question put in all innocence by a patient and guaranteed to drive the plastic surgeon insane is: 'If you're a plastic surgeon, that means you'll be using plastic, doesn't it?' At such a moment he may well regret ever having taken up the speciality and acquired such a title, for no plastic surgeon ever uses plastic derivatives and, indeed, prefers to avoid the use of foreign materials in adjusting shape and form wherever there are enough of the patient's own tissues to rearrange or transfer. In some cases, however, such as increasing the size of the breasts, the surgeon is grateful for the availability of one synthetic material – silicone. Silicone is biologically inert, can easily be sterilized, and takes on very different physical characteristics ranging from those of an oily liquid to those of a hard, solid block depending on its degree of chemical polymerization. Its consistency can therefore be selected according to need: in its soft form, for example, it is good for augmenting breasts, and in its solid state can be carved into a shape suitable for altering the profile of a nose, cheek-bone or chin. It is not, however, the perfect implant, as will become apparent in later chapters.

[5]

The Anaesthetic

Sometimes the fear of anaesthesia is so great that a patient will ignore even a serious disorder so as to avoid undergoing surgery and therefore general anaesthesia, hoping that it will somehow just 'go away'. Sadly, as a direct result of this dread, a disease or tumour that in the early stages might have proved amenable to rather less complicated treatment reaches a stage where a major and lengthy operation entailing far greater risks is called for; very rarely it may even become inoperable.

Not surprisingly, patients strongly motivated towards cosmetic surgery but with a terror of general anaesthesia prefer to live with their 'deformity', but if they do pluck up the courage to visit a cosmetic surgeon it is likely that they will ask more questions about the anaesthetic than about the surgery itself. No patient should feel ashamed or embarrassed to admit to this fear, and it may be of some consolation to know that many surgeons have the same reservations about undergoing surgery and general anaesthesia.

The medical profession does admit that the risk of death under general anaesthesia for all types of operations is about one in thirty thousand, and the occasional reports in the newspapers of death or failure to recover consciousness after an operation do nothing to allay one's fears. Such misgivings make it difficult to accept and find comfort in an account given by a surgeon of the efficiency and safety of a general anaesthetic, and it is only fair that a frightened patient should have a chance to talk at reasonable length with the anaesthetist, separately from the usual assessment and interview, before the operation so as to gain more knowledge and confidence.

Patients thinking of having a cosmetic operation should know that other forms of anaesthesia, such as local and 'twilight' anaesthesia, are also available; and in the USA, where much cosmetic surgery is performed in an office-type environment rather than in a traditional hospital, general anaesthetics are given less frequently than in Britain.

General Anaesthesia

Anaesthesia is defined as the loss of sensation, whether pain, pressure, heat or cold, and can be induced either in the whole body, by means of a general anaesthetic agent, or in a part, by a local one. For a patient to give a stranger, however well qualified, total control over his vital functions and to allow this person to make him unconscious and another to cut and refashion his flesh is an alarming prospect if one thinks carefully about it, and it is therefore right that a 'victim' should know something more of the background and training of an anaesthetist.

A common public misconception is that an anaesthetist is merely a technician who puts people to sleep and wakes them up again. The fact is that anaesthetists are fully qualified doctors who then opt to specialize in anaesthesia, just as other doctors choose to become general practitioners, cardiologists, pathologists, neurosurgeons or plastic surgeons. The training is long and comprehensive and meets very high standards, which are set and maintained by a national faculty of anaesthetists. Candidates are examined at various stages to assess their ability and, if successful, are given a certificate of accreditation which allows them to apply for a consultant post in anaesthetics. No one who fails any part of the specialist examination or who does not receive accreditation is eligible to be a consultant in the United Kingdom. A qualified anaesthetist is not only competent in all aspects of the subject relative to surgery, but is also expert in the relief of pain and in the management of the severely ill patient admitted to an intensive care unit; indeed, in many hospitals, anaesthetists run both the intensive care unit and their own pain-relief clinics. By dint of working almost daily together, the anaesthetist and surgeon eventually become a close-knit team with respect for each other's ability and mutual trust. Patients can overcome their own trepidation by putting the same trust in the ability and professionalism of the team.

Once the arrangements for admission have been made and the anaesthetist has been informed of the envisaged surgery, he will visit the patient before the operation to answer any queries, to win the patient's confidence and to make sure that anaesthesia proceeds smoothly. This is also the best time for the patient to air any worries or misgivings and for the anaesthetist to advise and reassure.

The interview and any tests cover three main aspects of the patient's health:

1. Habits and Physical Characteristics

The absorption, breakdown and excretion of anaesthetic agents depend on the efficiency of the lungs, heart, blood vessels, liver and kidneys, which can be impaired, for instance, by smoking, excessive alcohol intake, over-weight or allergic tendencies such as asthma and hay fever. Overeating is obvious on sight, but other habits and tendencies should be mentioned by the patient during the interview, as should any unpleasant or untoward reaction to previous anaesthetics and medication, such as a rash, sickness or nausea, since only if the anaesthetist has been made aware of any significant factors can steps be taken to prevent the occurrence of undesirable side-effects and incidents in the patient's sub-sequent treatment. In fact much of this sort of information can be obtained from hospital notes, but if the patient has moved from an area served by a different hospital or clinic, or come under the care of a different surgeon, it is important both to retrieve the original records and to question the patient directly about his medical history. Obviously where there are no records, the patient will be the only source of information.

2. Presence of Other Medical Conditions

The anaesthetist will also want to know of disorders and diseases which might have a bearing on the advisability of a general anaesthetic. These include diabetes, high blood pressure, chest and heart trouble, and kidney and liver diseases.

3. Taking of Regular Medication

Many drugs such as sedatives and antidepressants enhance, counteract or inhibit the action of commonly used anaesthetic agents, and the patient should inform the anaesthetist if he is taking any so that complications can be avoided. The contraceptive pill is one of various drugs that can lead to clotting of the blood in the veins (known as deep-vein thrombosis), and if a woman on the pill has not already discontinued it on the advice of her general practitioner or surgeon, precautions can be taken at the time of surgery to diminish the risk of this happening. The anaesthetist should also know if the patient is undergoing steroid treatment, as the dosage needs to be increased during surgery.

In fact, since most of the information relevant to anaesthesia is available in the form of previous correspondence or records of out-patient attendances and hospital admissions, the anaesthetist will not usually have to spend a long time at the bedside, and during the interview will be mainly concerned with making sure that nothing has been withheld by the patient or omitted from the hospital notes that is likely to affect the outcome of the operation. If, in the course of the interview or on the basis of the records, the anaesthetist becomes uneasy about some feature of the patient's health, the operation, if it is not urgent (as with cosmetic procedures), will be postponed until what is wrong has been put right. Obviously if the problem is insurmountable, the patient will quite rightly be advised against undergoing any sort of cosmetic surgery. Where the operation is of extreme urgency, however, as in a life-and-death situation, the anaesthetist, having consulted with the surgeon as to the advisability of proceeding, will more often than not take a calculated risk with the anaesthesia and let the surgery go ahead.

The first stage of general anaesthesia is premedication, the administration of a mixture of drugs which prepare the patient physically and mentally for the operation. One ingredient of the cocktail is a drug that dries up the secretions of the mouth, throat and lungs, thus preventing the anaesthetic gas and its irritant vapours from stimulating excessive fluid production in the lungs and so giving rise to possible complications. Similarly the withholding of food and drink in the four to six hours prior to premedication ensures that the stomach will be empty at the time of surgery and that nothing will be 'brought up' to spill into the lungs. The other ingredients are sedatives and tranquillizers which make the patient relaxed and drowsy, and which may even send him to sleep before arrival at the anaesthetic room. It is here that anaesthesia proper begins, with the injection into a vein of a small amount of a drug belonging to the barbiturate family (thiopentone is one) which causes the patient to drift smoothly and gently off to sleep in a matter of seconds. It is quite a pleasant sensation marked only by a cold feeling in the arm or a curious but not disagreeable taste in the mouth. The terror occasionally encountered in a patient of lying awake but paralysed on the operating table, the anaesthetic having failed to work properly, and thus of having to endure the operation in silent agony, is no longer well founded (although such instances did occur, if very rarely, in a previous era of anaesthetic technique).

The next thing a patient will know is 'coming round' on a bed or comfortable trolley in a recovery room just as though waking up after a deep sleep, the only difference being that the tongue and mouth will be abnormally dry and the throat possibly a little sore following the use of a tube passed through the mouth into the windpipe to facilitate breathing and anaesthesia. The patient may also be aware of a clear, narrow flexible tube transporting fluid into one of the veins of the hand or forearm. The purpose of this 'drip' is to replace body fluid or blood lost in the course of the operation and to compensate for the liquid that could not be taken before surgery, thereby avoiding an uncomfortable sensation of thirst and reducing the chances of nausea. In the meantime the nurses will be quietly reassuring and will give drugs to alleviate any unpleasant after-effects of the operation.

Back on the ward the patient will be allowed to sleep with the help of drugs to suppress any sickness or pain until more complete recovery, when he may become aware of a slight stiffness in the upper back or shoulders depending on the duration of the operation. This stiffness, which wears off after a day or two, is caused by the fact that, in positioning the patient on the firm surface of an operating table, the theatre assistant has to straighten and extend his neck a little for anaesthetic purposes and for easy access to the head, face or neck, should the surgeon be operating on those areas.

The premedication, induction for general anaesthesia and early moments of waking up can amount to a not unpleasant experience. It is only in the further stages of recovery that a patient may become more aware of uncomfortable sensations, all of which can, however, be satisfactorily treated. There is little to fear and even something to enjoy.

Local Anaesthesia

Most cosmetic operations, such as scar revision and excision of unsightly and unwanted skin lesions, are relatively minor procedures that do not merit full anaesthesia and can be safely and quickly performed under local anaesthesia, allowing a patient to leave hospital immediately.

The drug used to induce local anaesthesia is given by injection and within a very short time blocks the conduction of electrical impulses in a particular nerve, thereby totally numbing the area it supplies. As anyone knows who has had a local anaesthetic injection from a dentist, the process is reversible and normal sensation is restored after one to two hours. The anaesthetic solution can be given either by local 'infiltration', in which the small sensory nerves lying immediately beneath the injection site are deadened, or as a nerve 'block', whereby a single large sensory nerve is infiltrated in isolation to numb a large area. A dentist uses both of these techniques – infiltration anaesthesia for the upper teeth, when the injection is given in the tissues around the base of the tooth itself, and block anaesthesia for the lower teeth, when the needle is passed into a site at the back of the mouth. In the latter case not only do all the lower teeth lose their feeling but the sides of the tongue and chin as well.

Although an operation using local anaesthesia is usually only a minor one, it is essential, as in any operation, for risks to be eliminated as far as possible; and for this reason all the usual operating-theatre procedures and rituals are carefully observed. Unless previously warned about what to expect, the patient may find the experience a little bewildering. In the first place, he will be asked to change into a gown and then escorted into a small operating room where the surgeon, assistant and nurses will already be waiting, gowned, capped and masked to guarantee sterility of the operation, and surrounded by the usual paraphernalia of bright overhead lights, glistening stainless-steel trolleys, diathermy machine, suture racks, operating stools, etc. The patient will then be asked to lie on the operating table, at which point a nurse will apply a thin metal diathermy plate to his thigh, for reasons that have already been mentioned in the previous chapter. The operative site will be exposed and cleaned with cool wet swabs soaked in a sterilized solution before being isolated from the surrounding area by green towels, and the surgeon will lightly mark the site of the incision on the skin with a sterile pen and inject the local anaesthetic. This is not 'just a small prick': it is more than that and rather like a wasp sting, except that the stinging disappears within a few seconds. After two to five minutes the anaesthetic will have taken full effect and the surgeon, having warned the patient that he is about to start, will make the first incision.

Undergoing an operation under local anaesthesia in a minor operating theatre is a relaxing experience that can be made more pleasurable by playing suitable music on a radio or cassette-player. There is also the chance for staff to talk to the patient throughout the operation, which helps to distract attention and disperse apprehension about what is actually happening. Unlike the victim in a dental chair with a mouthful of instruments, fingers, metal sucker and water, the patient is able to converse intelligibly and ask and answer questions rather than communicate by means of a few gargled grunts.

At the end of the operation, with sutures and dressings in place, the patient returns to the cubicle to change, after which he may leave the hospital. If no drug was used other than the local anaesthetic, he can drive a car and, if need be, return to work on the same day, but once the anaesthetic has worn off the wound will be a little sore and mild pain-killing tablets may be required.

Twilight Anaesthesia

Facelift, rhinoplasty, eyelid reduction, breast augmentation and many other major cosmetic procedures can be done under local anaesthesia, but other drugs need to be used to relieve pain and anxiety. Some of these operations take from one to three hours to complete and it is asking too much of a patient to lie quiet and wide awake on the operating table for such a length of time, regardless of the wit and conversational talents of the surgeon and staff.

'Twilight' anaesthesia is a solution, and here premedication similar to that used prior to general anaesthesia ensures that the patient is sedated and drowsy by the time he is wheeled into the operating room, lifted on to the table and appropriately positioned. A drip is inserted into a vein in the arm through which drugs can be injected at intervals to maintain the state of drowsiness, and the operative site anaesthetized with a local anaesthetic, using a combination of infiltration and nerve-block techniques. The surgery can then begin.

The term 'twilight' anaesthesia derives from the state of the patient, who is not fully aware of all that is going on but not unconscious either, and describes a technique that requires training and considerable expertise on the part of a surgeon who chooses to take responsibility for the anaesthesia in addition to the surgery itself. The practice is fairly common among cosmetic surgeons in America, particularly in the flourishing private sector, where obviously costs incurred in maintaining and staffing a complete suite of rooms (usually comprising consulting rooms, operating theatre, recovery area, dressing station, nursing and rest rooms and accounts office) have to be kept to a minimum. Twilight anaesthesia is advantageous in this respect, obviating the need for the anesthesiologist, as this type of specialist is called in the USA, although the occasional surgeon is the happier for being able to call on one during an operation. The disadvantages include both the usual risks – all surgical office suites contain resuscitation equipment that is mandatory in the traditional context where general anaesthesia is used – and the fact that it takes time for the patient to recover from the effects of the analgesics and sedatives used to complement the local anaesthetic – sometimes more so than in recovering from a conventional general anaesthetic. In Britain, although cosmetic surgeons readily admit that they operate privately to make money, the majority are also committed to their work in the public sector and do not have the time, let alone the inclination, to run an office surgery system along American lines. In general, in this country, a cosmetic surgeon will operate on fee-paying patients in a private hospital, which is only a smaller version of the state-run kind, and have an anaesthetist present regardless of whether surgery is to be under twilight or full anaesthesia.

Although office surgery may not have caught on in this country, British surgeons have been influenced by the transatlantic trend of keeping patients in hospital for as short a time as possible. Not only does this allow more operations per week but it also gives patients the welcome chance to sleep in their own beds on the next or even the same day. As candidates for cosmetic surgery are on the whole physically fit they are ideally suited for short-stay surgery, and an increasing number of operations are now carried out under general anaesthesia as day cases. Indeed, some surgeons and anaesthetists believe that this type of anaesthesia allows the patient to return home in a more complete state of recovery than does twilight anaesthesia, although he must never leave unaccompanied and must always make arrangements to be met by a friend or relative and driven home.

Acupuncture

Acupuncture has been an integral part of traditional Chinese medicine for thousands of years and remains a proven form of treatment for many ailments in China. The interest of the Western world in acupuncture has also led to its adoption here, if only in the sphere of 'fringe medicine', and it is now acknowledged as being of value to many individuals whose problems have proved resistant to more conventional, 'scientific' practice.

Dramatic and convincing documentaries have been shown of Chinese patients smiling and laughing into the camera while undergoing major abdominal and chest surgery with the only evidence of anaesthesia being the acupuncture needles stuck into various parts of their anatomy, but closer investigation has shown that not all patients are in fact susceptible to the powers of acupuncture, just as not all patients respond to hypnosis. During a recent interview in China, leading surgeons admitted that acupuncture is so unpredictable a form of anaesthesia and, even if it works, takes so many hours to prepare that preference is generally given to the quicker and more reliable forms introduced from the West.

SURGICAL GAZETTEER

Introduction

A person taking a holiday or travelling in an unfamiliar country will usually make some sort of preparation for the trip, whether in learning about the regional characteristics of the area, its food and wines, or about any unusual diseases necessitating prior protection in the form of immunization, and will often try to learn a few words or phrases of the country's language that might be useful or add interest to the holiday. Booksellers are well aware of the needs of the occasional and professional traveller and make available a wide range of guide-books and maps for their use.

Yet the occasional patient (fortunately the professional patient is very rare) about to undergo surgery is often ill prepared for the experience. Wherever the fault may lie – with the surgeon who has not the time or patience to explain the operation or its possible outcome fully, with the patient who fails to understand the surgeon's explanation, or with the individual who has a blind, unquestioning faith in the 'miracle' of modern surgery – the surgical consumer does not often have a guide-book to unknown surgical territories. Handbooks explaining accepted cosmetic surgical procedures do exist, but they are not written by surgeons and therefore lack authenticity. The Surgical Gazetteer attempts to fill this gap.

The information in this section of the book is directed at patients who may need clarification on certain aspects of a particular cosmetic operation. Although it is based mainly on the personal experience of one surgeon, it also draws on the experience of other surgeons expert in particular procedures and on interviews with patients both satisfied and dissatisfied. The aim of the Gazetteer is to prepare a patient pre-operatively in terms of the general surgical technique, the pain or dis-comfort to be expected after the operation, the potential hazards, the anticipated immediate and long-term results, the time necessary for a return to work and normal life, and whatever personal adjustments will be called for. However, the reader should bear in mind that what follows is not a universally accepted code of cosmetic-surgical practice graven on tablets of stone: no two surgeons treat a patient in exactly the same way, and if, on reading this section, patients discover that their treatment differs from the text, they should not necessarily conclude that something is amiss but rather take into account that this is a purely personal account of cosmetic procedures, and one that cannot therefore be justifiably used to instigate, support or deny any claims for compensation on the grounds of negligent treatment.

Appendix A outlines how to set about looking for surgery in the United Kingdom, and describes the system of referral and pre-surgical preparation. Appendix B describes means available for redress in the rare event of a patient being confronted by a totally unsympathetic surgeon where there are reasonable grounds for complaint.

[6]

Scars

Most cuts in the skin, if properly managed, eventually form a fine but permanent line of scar tissue, a process that occurs as a result of a complex and ill-understood biological sequence of events. Erudite textbooks and papers abound on the subject, and national and international symposia on wound-healing attract hordes of high-flying scientists who meet to puzzle over the control of defect-repairing cells and tissues. A Nobel Prize certainly awaits the team that unravels this particular mystery, for not only will it be a major breakthrough in itself but it may also provide the key to the understanding and treatment of abnormal scar behaviour and abnormal cell behaviour in cancerous growths. In the meantime patients and surgeons must be content with a description rather than an understanding of events.

In the first three days after an operation an accurately sutured cut is filled with cells that secrete a 'cement' in the form of spirals of collagen fibres. The deposition of collagen is so brisk that it can join the edges of a wound together within a week, and it is at this point that the sutures are usually taken out. However, the new channels of microscopic blood vessels transporting the cells to the wound site give the fresh wound an abnormally red appearance that shows through the thin layer of epithelial cells or skin that has bridged the narrow gap, so that the newly forming scar will be both red and raised for some time after the removal of the sutures. Over the succeeding months, as the collagen matures and the tiny blood vessels involute, the scar flattens and fades until eventually only a fine white line remains. The same process occurs with a wound having a larger gap, but here the tissues have to contract before the usual sequence of biological repair can begin.

It is quite impossible for a surgeon to predict how long it will take a given scar to mature, the behaviour of a scar varying from individual to individual and from site to site; the best estimate he can give a patient is three to nine months. Similarly the surgeon cannot guarantee the final appearance of any scar, and even a 'normal' one may have certain unacceptable features after a year, such as bevelled edges, a central depression and cross-hatching caused by the sutures. Furthermore, in the earlier phase of collagen maturation a scar can sometimes contract (scar contracture is a totally different phenomenon from wound contracture), thereby causing distortion of adjacent tissues and structures. Both here and in normal scar development it is very important to allow full maturation to take place before undertaking any form of revision, for time is a great improver and can perform seeming miracles on even the ugliest scar. Not infrequently revision will be completely unnecessary, but even if further treatment is required at the end of the maturation period, it will be simpler and less extensive than would have been the case in earlier months. Thus surgeons do their best to persuade patients that it is not in their best interest to have their disfiguring scars repaired in the first few months after surgery, but that they should wait at least six months and let nature do most of the improving before thinking of surgical correction.

Abnormal Scars

1. *Hypertrophic Scars*

Sometimes a surgical incision beautifully repaired under ideal conditions develops into a scar lumpier and wider than is normal, forming an ugly red nodule or ridge and a source of intense frustration for the surgeon and distress for the patient. Hypertrophic scars, as they are called, are caused by an imbalance between collagen formation and collagen degradation, in which the result of the equation is too much collagen, and although they do eventually mature, by 'eventually' is implied at least two years, which is a long time for anyone to tolerate a lump that not only looks ugly but as a result of the brisk cellular activity within it is irritatingly itchy. Unfortunately there is no sure way of telling which individual will develop a scar of this kind, although burns and abrasions of intermediate skin depth predispose to hypertrophic scarring in young patients.

2. Keloid Scars

Another mystery, fortunately rarer than hypertrophic scarring, is the persistently over-active scar which generates so much abnormal collagen that it piles up into a tumour-like mass and spills over the margins of the repaired wound on to normal skin. A graphic description of the keloid scar, which is not only an eyesore but very difficult to treat effectively, is afforded by its name, which derives from the Greek *chele* for a crab's claw. Although keloid scarring cannot be foreseen there are certain sites that are more at risk than others, namely the central chest and sternal area, the upper outer shoulder, and the upper back. Surgeons try to avoid operating on these sites, but if compelled to do so warn patients of the possible consequences. Certain people are also more at risk, and individuals of African and Asian origin, unlike Caucasians, are especially prone to keloid scarring. Ear-piercing is a common contributory factor and often leads to the development of an unsightly mass behind the ear-lobe. This is not to say that every scar in every dark-skinned patient will be a keloid scar, but the danger is there.

3. Stretched Scars and Stretch-marks

Where a well-repaired and normally healed scar is subjected to constant stress the collagen fibres beneath the outer or epidermal layers of the skin rupture and separate along the axis of the greatest force. Thus, while the scar does not actually dehisce and break down it gradually widens to form a broad, flat white mark. As might be expected, sites particularly prone to this type of scarring are areas that are repeatedly subjected to stretching and bending movements; and patients should be warned that the removal of a lesion from any of these will usually lead to a stretched scar. It is very tempting to revise the latter, but the patient must accept that, although immediately after revision a nice thin line will form, it will inevitably begin to stretch again, however heavily the wound may have been surgically reinforced. It is true, however, that a revised stretched scar is often more acceptable than the original version.

Skin collagen can also rupture and separate in otherwise normal and previously uninjured skin to form striae better known as stretch-marks. During pregnancy, for example, the skin envelope encasing the swelling abdomen or breasts may stretch at points of weakness to leave numerous flat pale marks that will remain long after the birth of the baby. These are very difficult to treat except by excision, when redundant abdominal and breast skin is removed (see Chapters 16 and 17). Stretch-marks are seen not only in women after pregnancy but also in people who rapidly gain weight or who body-build themselves for athletic or exhibition purposes. Not all individuals acquire stretch-marks, of course, and it can be galling for a young woman following the birth of her first child to compare her own slack, stretched abdomen and breasts with those of an older woman who may have had several children yet who does not have a single stretch-mark or redundant skin fold. Such differences are inevitable given the variability of individuals' response to the stresses of nature, accident or disease.

4. Pigmented Scars

Scars are always different in colour from the surrounding skin, whether redder in the early phase of maturation or paler in the late, mature phase, but this is quite normal. Unacceptable variations can occur, however, and are caused, for example, by foreign materials such as road dirt or oil particles embedding themselves in the wound at the time of injury. The resulting scars are known as traumatically tattooed scars and can be effectively treated only by surgical revision. Undesirable differences in tone can also arise in dark-skinned people where the pigment cells at the base of a scar behave inappropriately and either fail to produce enough pigment, giving a pale or hypopigmented scar, or generate too much, leaving an abnormally dark or hyperpigmented scar. It is beyond the scope of any physician or scientist to control the behaviour of a pigment cell, so that patients have either to come to terms with the situation or opt for cosmetic camouflage.

How to Make Ugly Scars Less Ugly

The wording of the above heading may be harsh, but it serves to emphasize the inevitable truth that a scar is a scar is a scar, and that the permanent mark it leaves can never be made to look pretty, not even by the most ingenious surgeon. The following techniques are those most commonly encountered in scar revision.

1. *Surgical Revision*

The simplest and most effective method of scar improvement consists of excision of the scar and meticulous resuturing of the wound margins, and is used to treat 'normal' scars with unacceptable contour defects, hypertrophic scars, pigmented scars and stretched scars. In very special circumstances it is also used for keloid scars where other lines of treatment have failed, for although total excision of this scar will almost invariably lead to the formation of an even bigger keloid, intralesional excision (i.e., with a thin rim of scar tissue left behind) and careful resuturing will reduce the bulk of the keloid in the long term. Surgical scar revision is usually carried out under local anaesthesia, which allows the patient to be discharged from hospital the same day, and only if the scars are particularly extensive will a general anaesthetic sometimes be advised.

The revised scar, although far neater and less perceptible, will be a little longer than the original since the traces left by the sutures and extending beyond the actual scar are also removed. However, if the scar is additionally reorientated to fall into a natural creaseline, thus ensuring that it will not become lumpy or hypertrophic and, unhampered by abnormal stress forces, will form a thin line, it may even double in length, albeit in the form of a zigzag. This type of revision, which involves breaking up the line of a scar, is known as Z-plasty (see Fig. 1), W-plasty or multiple Z-plasty. In general the wound is sutured with a weaving stitch beneath its surface so as to avoid leaving suture marks, but if conventional sutures are used they will be removed at the earliest possible opportunity, usually after four or five days, and replaced with adhesive tapes. These will be left on for ten to fourteen days until the newly formed collagen is strong enough to support the wound margins without assistance. The revised scar will now have to pass through all the usual stages of maturation before a real improvement is seen: there is obviously no such thing as an instant transformation.

2. *Steroid Therapy*

The abnormal behaviour of collagen-producing cells within the hypertrophic and keloid scar can be moderated to some extent by means of steroids. Low doses are either injected directly into the scar by means of a needle and syringe, causing a sharp pain that wears off within minutes, or administered under high pressure in aerosol form, with

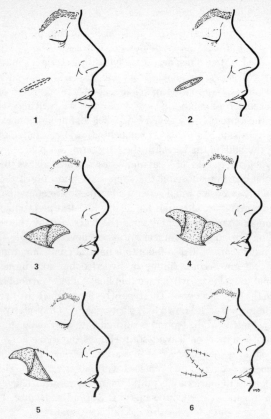

Fig. 1 An ugly scar lying in the wrong direction can be excised and re-orientated to follow a natural creaseline by means of a Z-plasty, leaving a longer but neater scar.

relatively little pain and accompanied by a somewhat startling noise like that of an airgun. Alternatively, steroid-impregnated adhesive tapes, cut to the shape of the scar, can be used with a fair degree of success to release steroid particles slowly into the skin and thus to flatten the scar over a period of months. The use of steroids for these two types of scars is empirical, but after a series of injections at intervals of four to six weeks most hypertrophic scars are paler, flatter and less itchy.

3. Dermabrasion

An air drill similar to the type dentists use can improve the irregular surface of a scar by smoothing it down, rather as in planing the rough contours of a crude wooden surface, and is also useful, in the case of pigmented scars, for removing particles embedded in the skin. Small areas can be done under local anaesthesia, but as the noise of the drill can be disturbing and the scars undergoing revision are usually on the face, it is more helpful to give a general anaesthetic, the patient in any case being discharged the same day. The freshly dermabraded area is tender and moist, and dressings have to be worn for up to ten days until the skin has regenerated. It may take several months for the new skin to take on a normal colour and during this time it will be pinker than its surroundings, like the skin that forms after a shallow sunburn. In this interval it should be kept well oiled with skin creams and, if desired, disguised with make-up.

4. Injectable Collagen

A new product has recently been introduced that can be used to fill out the depressions and furrows of wrinkles and repair the cavities and contour defects of normal and stretched scars. The material is collagen, taken from cows and purified in such a way that it can safely be injected into human skin, although since 2 per cent of patients show an allergic response to the substance a small preliminary test dose is essential. The main dose is deliberately over-injected into the scar, 60 per cent of the mixture being absorbed in the first few hours and therefore having to be discounted. The remaining collagen is also broken down, if only gradually, over the succeeding months, so that in order to maintain the desired effect further injections are usually required at intervals of four to eight months. Injectable bovine collagen provides only a temporary solution in the treatment of depressed scars and wrinkles, and it is to be hoped that a more reliable, biologically inert material will be available in the future.

5. External Pressure

The overproliferated collagen in lumpy, hypertrophic and keloid scars can be flattened with the help of tight, individually tailored garments that exert constant pressure on the affected area. As can be imagined, it is not easy to apply this treatment to the face or neck, although specially designed compressive masks are used in patients with extensive, ugly hypertrophic scars resulting from a total facial burn. It is easier to compress the overproductive scar on a surface such as the chest, but the patient must accept that for this technique to succeed the garment should be worn day and night for not less than six months and removed only for toilet purposes. Not surprisingly, few patients tolerate pressure treatment unless their scars are very ugly and extensive or unless all other lines of treatment have failed.

6. *Low-dose Radiotherapy*

A surgeon is growing a little desperate when he feels it necessary to call on a radiotherapist for help with a benign skin lesion, but as must by now be clear, the keloid scar is not a simple skin problem and sometimes only a course of low-dose radiotherapy, by itself or in combination with surgical excision, will do the trick and improve it.

7. *Skin Grafting*

The use of a skin graft to replace a scar is likewise almost an admission of defeat, as skin grafts themselves are like large scars, and it is the extensive and bulky keloid scar defying all other forms of treatment that again comes under consideration. Revision in this case involves excision of the scar and resurfacing of the resulting large central raw area and thin rim of scar tissue with a split-skin graft (see Chapter 7).

8. *Cosmetic Camouflage*

During the long months of scar maturation when the patient is naturally self-conscious about her appearance and eager to avoid attracting undue attention from relatives, friends and strangers, properly applied cosmetic creams and powders can help to solve the problem, and suitably toned make-up can also be used to good effect in disguising any residual marks left after natural maturation or surgical revision. Often the shop-assistant in the cosmetics department of a chemist or large store will give sound advice as to the appropriate make-up, but if not the British Red Cross provides an invaluable service in cosmetic camouflage through dermatology and plastic-surgery departments in NHS hospitals.

	Unwanted features of normal scars	Hypertrophic scars	Keloid scars	Pigmented scars	Stretched scars
Surgical revision	Yes	Yes	Very rarely	Yes	Yes
Steroid therapy	Rarely	Yes	Yes	No	No
Dermabrasion	Yes	No	No	Yes	No
Injectable bovine collagen	Yes	No	No	No	Yes
External pressure	No	Yes	Yes	No	No
Low-dose radiotherapy	No	No	Yes	No	No
Skin grafting	No	No	Yes	No	No
Cosmetic camouflage	Yes	Yes	No	Yes	Yes

Fig. 2 Summary of the methods described for treating scars.

[7]

Skin Grafts

One general misconception that must be laid to rest is that grafting remedies all known skin defects, and without leaving a mark. The reverse is nearer the truth – especially in the case of a split-skin graft, which is in fact used only to resurface extensive raw areas resulting from burns or the excision of a large skin tumour, and never to solve the more simple cosmetic problems. It is also not widely known that there are two types of skin graft, each with its own attributes and indications for use – the split-skin graft and the full-thickness graft.

Split-skin Grafts

In the split-skin graft, only a thin layer of skin is removed, leaving behind intact skin cells from which new skin can grow. The area from which the graft is taken, known as a split-skin donor site, heals very rapidly, as a result of which split skin can be harvested from the same place over an extended period in separate sheets sufficient to cover, for example, the whole of the face and neck. The instrument used for removing the graft is a long flat blade set at a particular distance from a metal roller, the gap between the knife edge and the roller determining the thickness of the graft (see Fig. 3).

Unfortunately, there are considerable cosmetic and functional disadvantages to a split-skin graft which restrict its use, and a surgeon uses split-skin grafting on the face only as a last resort. One of the drawbacks is that the cells responsible for scar-tissue formation between the graft bed and the undersurface of the graft are extremely active and, by occupying a much greater area than in the usual linear scar, correspondingly increase the degree of surrounding tissue distortion

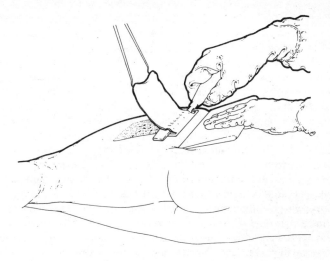

Fig. 3 A thin sheet is cut from the outer layer of the skin with a graft knife as a partial-thickness or split-skin graft. The raw bed heals by itself to form a pale patch.

secondary to graft contracture. The contractile force governing the graft is both powerful and relentless and can even overcome antagonizing muscle forces, with the result that the graft takes on a folded and wrinkled appearance, particularly in areas that normally have a wide range of movement such as the face or around a joint. Since it contains few elastic or normal collagen fibres, the graft also fails to stretch and relax like normal skin. This rigidity is obvious on the face of a badly burned patient where the grafted areas are expressionless and mask-like, contrasting with any unburnt, normal skin that remains.

Hopefully, armed with the knowledge gained thus far of the properties of a split-skin graft, a patient will not press a surgeon for this form of treatment; but there are yet more disadvantages. Elements normally present in the skin such as sweat glands, sebaceous glands and hair follicles are inevitably absent from this type of graft, which, when finally consolidated, will thus be dry, smooth, shiny and hairless. If it is used on the face it will also tend to be darker than the surrounding skin, as well as lacking the blush characteristics of normal facial skin.

Not only are there considerable cosmetic drawbacks to the skin graft itself, but also disadvantages at the donor site, which, having been stripped of its usual protective layer of skin, is particularly painful: after an operation the patient does not complain so much of pain in the resurfaced area as of stinging in the donor site, a sensation which however wears off after two or three days. Since the donor site bleeds, it has to be occluded with a bulky absorbent dressing, which is left on for ten to fourteen days until the skin has regenerated. The newly healed and exposed donor site is pink and tender, and requires daily attention in the form of gentle lavage and application of skin creams until it has matured, leaving an area marginally paler than the surrounding skin. In other words, a donor site forms a scar, and it is for this reason that graft skin is usually taken from areas that can be concealed, such as the buttocks or upper thighs.

For a skin graft to take, three things must be avoided – infection, movement between the graft and its bed, and accumulation of blood and serum at the graft/bed interface. To achieve this end, the surgeon covers the graft with a bulky sterile dressing impregnated with a suitable antiseptic solution, tying this over with sutures to provide pressure and thus to prevent both the formation of a space beneath the graft and sideways shift of the latter. The grafted area is then immobilized, where necessary (as with a wrist, elbow or knee) with a plaster-of-paris splint. The tie-over dressings and any splints are removed after seven to ten days, exposing what can often provoke horror even in the most carefully primed patient – understandably so, for a new skin graft has a staring, purplish-red discoloration and unsightly patches of crusts and blisters. However, these are easily removed by simple lavage and cream treatment over the succeeding days, and an intact, if discoloured, surface is soon obtained. As the graft matures and consolidates it gradually loses its bright colour until, after several months, it has assumed all the properties that identify a split-skin graft.

Full-thickness Skin Grafts

The full-thickness skin graft has totally different characteristics from the split-skin graft and, unlike the latter, whose use is avoided as far as

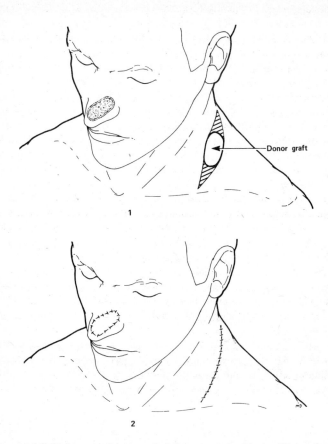

Fig. 4 A full-thickness graft leaves a bed that cannot heal by itself (1) and must be closed to form a linear scar (2).

possible, can reasonably be used in cosmetic surgery. However, this graft has the disadvantage that when it is removed from the donor area, a bed of muscle or fat is left from which new skin cannot possibly grow, and which must therefore be surgically closed like any other deep wound (see Fig. 4). It follows from this that the size of the graft depends very much on whether or not the donor site can be directly sutured.

63

The advantage of the full-thickness graft lies precisely in its thickness, which is significant in that the thicker a graft the less abundant the scar tissue it forms and therefore the less pronounced its contracture – a major bonus when it is used on the face. More important where thickness is concerned, this type of graft retains all the normal skin elements, including the full complement of collagen and elastic fibres which impart natural movement and elasticity to the skin and thus to the graft once it has been transposed, as well as the glands and hair follicles, whose presence ensures that the graft will preserve its original texture in the new site. This obviously means that a surgeon has to be very careful in selecting donor skin for a given area. Clearly it is not in a male patient's interest to have bearded neck skin taken over to the forehead, although on the other hand the property of a full-thickness graft in transporting hair is a distinct advantage in the treatment of baldness.

The donor sites commonly used in resurfacing small areas on the face are the base of the neck, the back of the ear and, in older individuals, the upper eyelid (in which case patients have the added benefit of an eyelid reduction), since skin taken from above the level of the collar-bone, as well as being similar in colour to the face, also has the ability to undergo dynamic colour change, whether in suntanning or in blushing, and is thus particularly appropriate for facial use. This is not always the case with skin from below the collar-bone, which tends to be fixed in colour and darker than the face.

The management of a full-thickness graft is identical to that of a split-skin graft and its appearance immediately after removal of the dressings equally unattractive, but there the similarity ends, for this type of graft can be a definite asset in cosmetic surgery when judiciously used.

[8]

Birthmarks and Skin Tumours

By far the most common of all cosmetic surgical operations is the removal of an unwanted skin lesion, whether a nodule, cyst or birthmark.

The skin is a very complex structure and it is not surprising that blemishes in the shape of birthmarks arise in the course of its formation. Comparable imperfections occur in the embryological development of other organs such as the liver, intestines and lungs, but unless they give rise to symptoms experienced by the patient they go unnoticed, uninvestigated and untreated, and it is only because of the unattractive appearance of a birthmark in the skin and the undesirable attention it may attract that a patient or a parent will seek medical advice.

Several types of birthmark can be distinguished, but those most often seen are brown birthmarks and red birthmarks, each with their own characteristics.

Brown Birthmarks

Everyone has at least one small brown mole on their skin, very often raised above the surrounding surface and carrying hairs. Most people do not worry about such blemishes and consider them part of their identity, physical traits to be usefully included in the section of a passport reserved for distinguishing features, if not actually to be regarded as beauty marks.

If a mole is ugly or excessively hairy, however, it is quite understandable that an individual may wish to have it removed, and there is no problem here providing the patient understands that he will instead acquire a scar that will obviously be just as permanent as the mole itself. Whether a scar is preferable to the mole or not is obviously the patient's matter," but he must realize before making any decision that the scar will be

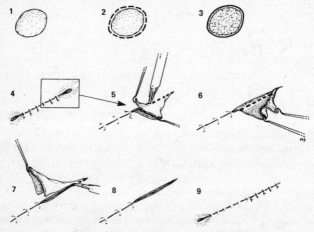

Fig. 5a When an incision is too small in relation to the original lesion (2), 'dog ears' appear at the ends of the wound (4) that have also to be excised (5–9).

much longer than he may have assumed, for if the surgeon were to remove nothing but the mole, an ugly, prominent 'dog ear' would appear at each end of the repair (see Fig. 5a). For this to be avoided, the length of the incision, and thus of the scar, must be roughly three times the diameter of the mole, which means that two triangles of normal skin are inevitably removed within the excised ellipse of skin containing the mole (see Fig. 5b). Skin grafts cannot be used to replace small moles removed for cosmetic purposes, for reasons that have already been mentioned in Chapter 7.

Occasionally a brown mole becomes disturbingly active, increasing in height or growing into the surrounding skin like a spreading ink-blot.

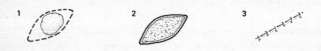

Fig. 5b If excision is to result in a neat scar, the length of the cut must be roughly three times the diameter of the lesion.

This phenomenon is quite natural in young children, particularly around puberty, and also in pregnancy, but if parents are worried about their child in such an instance, the surgeon will generally be willing to remove the mole (easily done under local anaesthesia) and ask the pathologist to examine the specimen under the microscope in order to verify its innocence. Innocence is assumed because, whereas the reasonable concern of the parents stems from their fear that the child's rapidly growing mole may be cancerous, a malignant melanoma (the term used for a cancerous brown lesion) is exceedingly rare in childhood and in fact only a few reports have been published in the literature worldwide. Unfortunately this is not the case in adult life, where any abnormal activity in a mole requires urgent attention. The changes here may of course simply be part of the benign process seen in childhood, but in any case it is essential to make certain that they are not in fact of a malignant nature. The pathologist is the only person who can confidently make this diagnosis, and does so by means of a biopsy, which is the examination of material removed from the living body – in this case of the mole itself. In the first instance, the mole is excised within the usual ellipse as the pathologist's specimen. If it subsequently proves to be malignant, a large area of skin surrounding the original site is also removed in order to provide adequate clearance and thus to check the sinister growth. This may seem a drastic treatment, and it is very distressing for a patient to be told that an area of skin roughly the size of a hand has to be removed for a 'spot', but a malignant mole, like any other form of cancer, is extremely dangerous and the surgeon has no choice in the matter, however much he may dislike excising such a large piece of skin and leaving a scarred, concave defect that is the inevitable long-term result of resurfacing the site with a split-skin graft. Under these circumstances, however, proper treatment of the cancer is essential and cosmetic compromises cannot be risked.

The large brown birthmark occurs less frequently than the mole, but this is no comfort to the individual who happens to be disfigured by a dark, hair-bearing patch that may extend over much of the body or, worse still, over half the face or neck. Even if the mark is in a place that is usually covered, occasions will inevitably arise when it will cause its owner considerable embarrassment and distress (one might here recall the sad example of the Indian wolf-boy who was covered entirely by a dark, hairy birthmark and who as a result was treated as a freak and exhibited in fairs). The pigment in this type of birthmark reaches deep into the skin, so that excision needs to be extensive, comprising even the subcutaneous layer of fat.

The skin graft used to cover the wound has all the usual cosmetic and functional disadvantages, but these are often deemed preferable to a disfigurement of this kind. However, as an alternative to the grafts already described, a method exists whereby a full-thickness flap of skin is raised from a part of the body adjacent to the wound and, still attached along one side or by a pedicle to its original bed, which ensures that blood vessels will continue to enter and feed it, is turned so as to cover and eventually grow into the raw area. The secondary wound left in the donor site is then closed. Needless to say additional scars are introduced, but this is a fair exchange for the original mark and preferable to a skin graft.* Unfortunately it is impractical to graft completely the very extensive brown birthmark covering the whole of the trunk, back and abdomen, and only if the patient finds life utterly intolerable in this respect will a staged surgical programme of excision and grafting be planned, with suitable intervals left for the graft to consolidate after each stage. Such a programme usually takes several years to complete.

It has recently been discovered, quite by chance, that in the first few weeks after birth the pigment of a giant brown birthmark lies only in the topmost layers of the skin, not yet having penetrated further. Happily this means that excision is unnecessary, and that the mark can be removed by surgical planing. It is not easy for a parent to accept the necessity of any operation so early in the life of a baby, but the results of dermabrasion at this stage are so promising as to be quite justifiable. The cells producing the pigment move to the deeper layers of the skin within a few months, so that the timing of the operation is critical.

Cancer is sometimes feared particularly by patients with a large brown birthmark, and although it is true that a malignant melanoma can develop in such a mark, it can equally well arise in a simple mole or even in an area of skin previously free from unusual pigmentation. In fact there is no convincing evidence that a large birthmark has a significantly greater risk of becoming malignant, but once the fear is raised

* A description of the many types of flaps available to a plastic surgeon is beyond the scope of this book, although the hair-bearing scalp flap will be dealt with in the chapter on baldness and some others in the chapter on breast surgery. If a flap is proposed it is better to discuss the relevant techniques, rationale and potential complications directly with the surgeon concerned.

reassurance is not always sufficient, and where possible the mark should be removed and examined by the pathologist. The process is much the same as for the disquietingly active mole, and here again biopsy provides the most reliable diagnosis.

Red Birthmarks

Red birthmarks owe their colour to the fact that they consist of a mass of dilated blood vessels. Many varieties are described, with differences in the site and appearance of the mark and also in the type and distribution of the blood vessels, but for the purposes of the patient two main groups can be distinguished – the diffuse, flat red mark occurring predominantly on the face and neck with a fixed, even colour and known as a port-wine stain, and the soft, spongy, red-speckled swelling called a strawberry mark, which can crop up anywhere.

1. Port-wine Stains

The port-wine stain, which is seen at birth and which can cover any part and extent of the face and neck, is due to the presence of a tightly knit network of fine capillary vessels in the superficial, intermediate or deep layers of the skin. The precise level of the network is significant as it influences the line of treatment, so as a preliminary and to establish the character of the stain, the surgeon asks the pathologist to examine a small piece of affected skin taken from the patient under local anaesthesia. If the stain is superficial its appearance can generally be improved by diathermy or laser therapy, but it must be acknowledged that there is as yet no completely satisfactory method of treating a port-wine stain whatever its depth.

According to recent reports, the argon laser gives the best results for the shallow type, but a comparable effect can be achieved by literally burning off the superficial layer of skin with a surgical diathermy blade and allowing it to heal naturally over the succeeding weeks. Whether the laser or the more economical diathermy technique is used, an acceptable outcome is seldom the case with a single session, and several are needed to build up the improvement and finally achieve an acceptably pale surface. Neither technique is as predictable with the intermediate type of stain and, indeed, both are relatively ineffective with the deep-seated complex, so in these two cases the surgeon may have to excise the whole depth of the stain and cover the wound with a skin graft or flap.

One other technique, derived from the tattooist's art, is occasionally tried. Here, with the help of suitable instruments, a paste of pale pigment is driven into the stain which, in blending with the colour imparted to the skin by the fine capillaries, produces a tone relatively similar to that of the surrounding skin. To use the patient's face like an artist's palette may seem a little strange, but dramatic improvements can be achieved, and even though the pigment does tend to leach out over the years, the colour of the skin remains less vivid and can be obscured reasonably well with light make-up. Properly applied cosmetics are in fact the most common treatment for a port-wine stain, although men are usually less enthusiastic about their use than women.

2. *Strawberry Marks*

An abnormal collection of larger veins and arteries usually extending into the deeper tissues of the skin is responsible for the strawberry mark. Although present at birth, complex structures of this type, when they occur, may not become apparent for some time, since it is only after an interval of several weeks to two months, during which the baby's circulatory mechanism becomes more established, that the blood vessels fill, producing the characteristically stained, soft swelling. The sudden appearance of an ugly red lump in the skin of an otherwise healthy baby can naturally perplex and worry its parents, but these swellings are in fact among the commonest in infancy and are entirely benign.

The occurrence of a strawberry mark is one of the many occasions where nature is the best physician, for in the natural course of events the swelling, after distending to greater dimensions and even intensifying in colour up to the age of one year, usually then begins to shrink and finally vanishes. What actually causes the disappearance is the fact that the flow of blood within the complex, being abnormally sluggish, gradually clots and blocks off the veins, undergoing a process very similar to that seen in the progressive silting up of a winding, slow-flowing stream. The usual policy is therefore non-intervention, and, as a rough guide, 20 per cent of these birthmarks will have resolved spontaneously by the age of two, 30 per cent by the age of three, 40 per cent by the age of four, and so on. However, 10 per cent of birthmarks remain, and in this case, particularly if they constitute a nuisance, are generally excised.

Surgery is also useful for tidying up the unsightly sac of thin redundant skin that may remain after total natural resolution of a bulky strawberry mark.

Nodules, Cysts and Patches

The protective skin envelope is the largest human organ and, as an external layer, susceptible to all manner of injuries, including those which can induce cell changes and thus lead to the formation of a skin tumour, whether harmless (benign) or harmful (malignant).

Because they are on the surface and thus apparent to the eye, skin tumours are usually noticed at an early and, in consequence, easily treatable stage of their development, and a patient who is conscious of their potential danger will more often than not immediately consult the doctor. This kind of self-diagnosis is of course impossible with internal organs, where a tumour may become quite large before being perceived, and even then can only be examined with the aid of X-rays or illuminated surgical telescopes. If the lining of the stomach could be scrutinized as easily and as frequently as the skin, the treatment of stomach tumours would undergo dramatic improvement, if only because of early detection. In any case, once they have become aware of it, owners of a new or growing skin lesion generally request its removal, either because they dislike the look of it or because they are worried that it might be cancerous. In the first place, therefore, and as with the suspect birthmark, the nodule, cyst or patch will be excised along with as little normal skin as possible and examined under the pathologist's microscope. If it proves to be benign, no further treatment will be necessary and the wound will eventually form a thin, neat scar. If malignant, however, as much skin will be removed from around the site as is deemed necessary to limit recurrence of the cancerous tumour. Where the subsequent wound cannot easily be closed it will be resurfaced either with a skin graft, preferably full-thickness, or with an adjacent skin flap.

[9]

Tattoos

The human instinct for self-decoration is apparent at all levels and in all types of society, and is expressed in an almost infinite number of ways. Among the most extreme of these, and certainly the most painful, is deliberate mutilation of the skin. Whatever the origin and nature of the mutilation, and whether it is a tribal scar or a professional naval tattoo, its purpose is generally the same: to declare identity or allegiance and thus to establish a bond with peers.

Allegiances change, however, and while an individual may easily discard a club tie in favour of another, or a fiancée return an engagement ring, it is not quite so simple for an ex-prison inmate to rid himself of a tattoo which identifies him for ever as having belonged to that institution or for a girl to remove a tattoo from her forearm which signifies attachment to a discarded boyfriend. To make matters worse, since many tattoos later regretted are acquired as a result of episodes that are viewed with disfavour by the general public – such as a wild adolescent party, a period of heavy drinking, flirtation with drugs, or membership of a group that is considered as undesirable or offensive – society quite often adopts a 'holier than thou' attitude to tattooed individuals, and there are sadly a few surgeons who actually refuse under any circumstances to remove tattoos. To the moralizing of such people is added the unfortunate misconception, with all its connotations of prejudice, that tattoos are somehow indicative of social and mental inferiority – a suggestion certainly not borne out by the facts.

If an individual decides for one reason or another, whether social pressure or personal preference, to have a tattoo removed (and only a minority actually take this step), it is important for him to realize that it is impossible to remove a tattoo without leaving a permanent scar in its place. The scar itself will vary according to the extent, depth and site of the tattoo, and this itself will depend to a large degree on whether the latter is of professional or amateur origin.

The professional tattoo is created by driving variously coloured salts into the skin with the aid of a hand-held motor-driven machine supplied with a head of multiple reciprocating needles, and although the process is accompanied by the same risk of pyogenic (pus-generating) infection and particularly of hepatitis as in the amateur type, it is safeguarded by the enforcement of standards that ensure sterility. The tattooist's fee is in proportion to the scale, intricacy and colouring of the design, which can be extremely complex and cover much of the body, as in the well-known example of a fox-hunting scene beginning on the lower abdomen, continuing up the chest and over the shoulder, and running down the back to follow the fox to ground between the buttocks. In general, the professional tattoo is more extensive and finer in execution than the less complicated and often rather crude amateur tattoo, which is usually applied with an ordinary needle using an easily available black pigment such as indian ink, graphite or mascara. This method, with its use of a simple needle, has the disadvantage that the pigment cannot be distributed evenly through the skin, so that the depth of the tattoo will tend to vary between the superficial layers of the skin and the fat or muscle beneath them. Such differences in the making of a tattoo obviously have a large bearing on the method of removal and its degree of success.

Everything from vinegar and stronger acids to stale urine and pigeon's excrement has been used over the ages in an attempt to remove tattooed pigment from the skin, and even today the professional tattooist will some-times apply nitric or sulphuric acid to an unwanted tattoo, with grim results. There is still no ideal treatment, but four established methods are used, each with its own indications, advantages and disadvantages.

Surgical Excision

Cutting out the tattoo remains the most common treatment, and one that guarantees complete removal of the pigment. The process is most effective with small tattoos, which can be excised directly and the wound sutured, leaving a straight or curved scar that attracts considerably less attention than the original design. The operation is performed under local anaesthesia and the patient sent home on the same day, the sutures being removed after the usual interval. Treatment for multiple small tattoos may require several sessions, but is equally simple.

Surgical Gazetteer

With a large tattoo it is usually impossible to close the wound directly, and, after the surface of the skin has been shaved off in layers with a graft knife until no pigment remains, one of two things can happen. If the tattooed particles occurred only in the superficial or intermediate layers of the skin, the deep layer that remains is allowed to heal spontaneously like a split-skin donor site (see Chapter 7), leaving a pale, flat scarred surface whose shape will give no indication as to the origin of the scar. If the pigment occupied the deepest layers (invariably the case with an amateur tattoo, and sometimes with the over-enthusiastic professional kind), a split-skin graft is used to cover the raw bed left after the required deep shaving, since it does not have the potential to generate new skin. The use of a split-skin graft entails all the usual disadvantages, but the long-term results of this traditional treatment in sites such as the arms or legs can be more satisfactory than those achieved with the more recent laser method. The whole tattooed area can be removed in one operation under general anaesthesia with the patient discharged on the same day, and the dressings protecting the skin graft and its donor site are removed after ten to fourteen days.

It is not in the patient's best interests to attempt complete removal of tapestry-type tattoos such as the fox-hunting scene, since apart from the scars being unacceptably extensive the excision of so much skin can be hazardous.

Dermabrasion

The use of high-powered air-driven instruments driving a small rotary wheel coated with diamond or carborundum particles has already been described in the removal of coloured fragments embedded in a wound during an accident. The sandpaper principle at work in the treatment of these traumatically tattooed scars applies equally in that of decorative tattoos, and specifically of those in the professional category, where the pigment has not been driven deep into the skin, and is particularly advantageous for surfaces that are difficult to shave with a skin-graft knife, such as the face or breasts.

Depending on its extent, the tattoo is dermabraded under local or general anaesthesia with the patient treated as a day case, but either way requires more than one session for the pigment to be completely removed. Even after several treatments, carried out at intervals of three to six months, residual pinpoints remain within the scarred area, giving

74

a ghost image of the original tattoo. These can be obliterated by means of selective surgical excision. The dermabraded area also has the disadvantage of being different in colour from the surrounding skin.

Salabrasion

Salabrasion is nothing new. In the sixth century AD, Aetius of Amida, court physician to Justinian I, wrote a mammoth work in sixteen volumes, the *Tetrabiblos*, in which, among some surprisingly innovative surgical procedures, he described the application of salt to the skin as a treatment for unwanted tattoos. This ancient technique is widely used today and is particularly suitable for the shallower professional tattoos acquired in the armed services. A paste of table-salt and sterile water is smeared over the tattoo and then rubbed into the surface with a sterile brush or piece of gauze until a raw surface is obtained. As rubbing salt into a wound is an uncomfortable experience, the area is either locally anaesthetized by means of the infiltration technique, or an anaesthetic cream is incorporated in the salt mixture. The dressing applied to the treated surface is removed about ten days later together with any loose scabs, leaving a partly depigmented tattoo and, curiously, a faded imprint of the tattoo, almost like a transfer, on the underside of the dressing. The treatment is repeated at three-month intervals until sufficient pigment has been removed.

Salabrasion is not the ideal solution, and is similar to dermabrasion in that a ghost tattoo remains within a faintly scarred area. However, a treatment of salabrasion followed immediately by dermabrasion is proving to have marginally better results than salabrasion alone.

Laser Therapy

The publicity given to the laser and its high-powered science-fiction image mislead quite a number of patients into thinking that laser therapy is *the* modern panacea, replacing all other lines of treatment – however simple, cheap and efficient – for tumours, eye diseases, effects of ageing, birthmarks and tattoos. In fact, although the laser is a welcome innovation, it is suitable for treating only a very few problems, one of these being the unwanted tattoo. Here the laser can certainly play an important part, while not entirely replacing other methods, and if a suitable type is available in a hospital or clinic it can reasonably be used to obliterate a tattoo. If not, the alternative methods described can be just as effective.

The carbon dioxide (CO_2) and ruby lasers have hitherto been most widely used for tattoo excision. Both successfully vaporize the ink but do not, as is frequently supposed, leave the skin wholly intact. In fact, there is skin destruction enough to leave a permanent scar, although the effects of the ruby laser are often less marked in this respect than those of the CO_2 laser. It is not a painless process, so a local anaesthetic is essential, and the lasered area, being raw and tender like a dermabraded or salabraded surface, is left covered with a post-operative dressing for about fourteen days until the skin has healed. Although it is impossible to remove the tattoo completely in one session and further treatments are needed at intervals of three months, all the pigment can undoubtedly be removed in time. The only disadvantage is that the patient is left with a permanent pale scar that can easily be identified as a treated tattoo unless the operator deliberately lases beyond the borders of the original design to produce a more amorphous patch resembling the mark left by a burn.

[10]

Surgery for Baldness

Nineteen out of twenty men suffer some degree of hair loss and, not surprisingly, hair transplantation has become the most common cosmetic operation in males. Balding is in most cases a completely normal, natural phenomenon which is at the same time extremely variable in extent and type, ranging from almost undetectable thinning and recession of the hairline at the forehead to virtual absence of all hair. The time of onset is also subject to variation: one can remember senior boys at school whose hair was already and quite noticeably beginning to recede.

Alopecia, as baldness is known, normally occurs as a result of genetic predisposition (i.e., it is hereditary) combined with the influence of male hormones, called androgens, on the hair follicles, and is not, as is widely believed, due to an excess of male hormones and thus a sign of greater virility. By the same token, a full head of hair is not a mark of effeminacy associated with a lack of androgens but a hereditary trait: a man with insignificant hair loss is likely to have a father, grandfather and uncles who all, like him, have a thick, full mane of hair and who yet have a normal complement of male hormones. Occasionally, balding can be a symptom of disease, and as such is considered a pathological (abnormal) phenomenon rather than a physiological (normal) one. Here the priority is naturally treatment of the disease itself rather than of the sign of the disease, and correct diagnosis is essential. Fortunately, most practitioners of hair-transplant surgery are well qualified to distinguish between normal and abnormal baldness. More rarely, temporary alopecia can also be caused by certain drugs, chemicals and therapies, and some affections of the skin can also damage the hair.

The principle governing surgery for male baldness is the redistribution of whatever scalp hair the patient has remaining and, more particularly, its transfer from the sides and back of the head to the denuded areas high on the forehead and on the dome. In this process, the total number of hair follicles on the scalp remains unchanged, although the bulk of the hair can be increased by growing it to a longer length. Transplantation of hair obtained from sites other than the patient's scalp has been tried but found wanting, as hair from the armpits, chest and pubic region has characteristics which distinguish it quite clearly from scalp hair and which therefore make it look quite out of place when transferred to the head. An alternative method consists of actually weaving artificial or trimmed human hair into the scalp. This is harmful as well as pointless, and it is far more sensible to wear a wig or toupée of human hair than to thread the strands into the skin itself.

By no means all men find normal balding unacceptable enough to warrant surgery, and only a small percentage in fact seek to enhance their image by correcting what they regard as a premature and un-desirable sign of ageing. Individuals who do decide in favour of treatment should consult a recommended practitioner or surgeon rather than answer the call of an advertisement in a magazine, newspaper or railway station, as clinics that publicize themselves in this way are not always to be trusted. They should also be prepared for a refusal on the part of the surgeon to operate, as not all men are suitable candidates for correction of baldness. Prospective patients who have been refused treat-ment should accept the verdict rather than embark on a hunt for a 'tame' hair-transplant surgeon, since, even if in the end they do find someone willing to perform surgery, they are likely to be even more demoralized by the outcome than by their original condition.

Unsuitable patients include those with extensive balding and therefore insufficient hair for a useful transplant, those with very scanty and thinly distributed hair, and those with fine blond hair, in whom the results will never be satisfactory. If there is dermatitis or infection of the scalp, surgery is definitely contra-indicated, while patients with dark skin should be aware of the risk of ugly, hypertrophic or keloid scarring (see Chapter 6).

The ideal candidate is healthy, well motivated, aged between twenty-five and fifty, with thick dark hair and a relatively stable area of baldness affecting the front and top of the scalp. However, even this type of patient should realize that a full, bushy head of hair can never be achieved and that, while the bald sites can be resurfaced, any improvement is at the expense of the hair-bearing areas.

Baldness in women is a far less frequent occurrence than in men, and when it does arise takes the form of general thinning rather than loss from a specific and therefore more noticeable area. Appropriate hair-styling is usually enough to disguise any defects, although if the alopecia is severe, a hair transplant can be performed. The procedure is exactly as for men, and makes use either of hair-bearing skin grafts or of, flaps, according to the technique.

Hair-bearing Grafts

The donor area on the side or back of the head is trimmed and cleaned and then injected with a solution containing local anaesthetic and adrenalin, which as well as anaesthetizing the area also reduces bleeding. The recipient site is similarly prepared, following which a sterile metal punch with sharp edges is used to remove cylinders of hair-bearing skin from the donor site. Experience has shown that a cylinder measuring more than 4.0 mm across has a less predictable take after transfer than is desirable, so the usual diameter is 3.5–4.0 mm, while the depth of the cylinder is such as to include intact and viable hair follicles. What is involved here is thus a full-thickness rather than a partial-thickness graft. The punch is then used to excise cylinders of bald skin from along the forehead, thus making room for the grafts and creating a natural hairline with a slightly irregular margin and a widow's peak. The excised skin is discarded and the hair grafts implanted in their new sites, oriented in such a way as to leave the hair follicles pointing in the direction of normal hair growth (see Fig. 6). The raw donor sites are allowed to crust over and will have healed completely by the end of a fortnight. Occasionally, if the donor sites bleed excessively, sutures are used to stop the flow. These are removed one week later.

An alternative method uses hair-bearing strips with a width of 6 mm and a length of up to 8 cm as the starting point for a new frontal hairline. This technique has the advantage of transferring a greater number of hair follicles in a single graft than is possible with a punch graft, but is complicated by the fact that it is technically more difficult and has a higher risk of incomplete hair growth. Sometimes a strip graft has such patchy results that it has later to be augmented with punch grafts. In fact, many practitioners now prefer a combination of grafts, using strip grafts to form the new hairline and backing these up with punch grafts distributed over the dome and remaining scalp. Ten to fifty punch grafts and one strip graft are usually transferred in one session. Other sites can

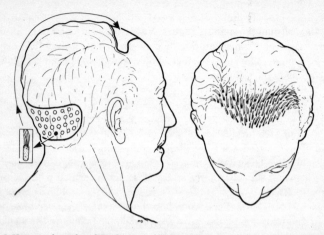

Fig. 6 Hair can be redistributed using cylindrical hair-bearing punch grafts taken from the back and sides of the head and 'seeded' in the frontal bald area.

be grafted later, but a patient must be prepared to wait at least three months between each treatment session, surgery being repeated until a reasonable distribution of hair has been achieved or until no more hair can be removed from the donor sites.

Whatever the method, a head bandage is worn for the first three days after the operation to protect and immobilize the grafts, and in the week following its removal the patient is advised not to wash his hair and to take care when brushing or combing the established hair to avoid touching the grafts. Some discomfort at both the donor and recipient sites is to be expected during this time. The patient must not look for an instant improvement, and should discount any initial growth of hair from the grafts, since this is a false spurt heralding complete loss of the newly implanted hair at four weeks. In fact the hair follicles have to go through a resting or recuperative phase lasting three months before they can start to generate hair once more, and even then growth is slower than usual, amounting to no more than half an inch per month, so that the patient has to wait at least six months to a year before seeing the final results. In the meantime he should also expect the surface of the punch grafts to have a slightly cobbled appearance, and should be prepared for patchy numbness of the scalp where the necessarily deep embedding of the graft may have damaged a small nerve. This is only a temporary effect, however, and depending on the extent of the injury, normal sensation will have returned after six to eighteen months.

The procedure of transplanting hair-bearing grafts has been compared with the returfing of a lawn, but a lawn prepared in this way gives an almost instant result with no easily detectable gaps. In fact the process is more akin to the planting of a herbaceous border, in that the small, widely separated plants look sadly isolated and sparse in the late spring but burgeon and flourish over the months to provide an attractive, matted bed of flowers by the end of the summer.

Hair-bearing Flaps

In the last ten years or so, surgeons specializing in the treatment of baldness have taken a growing interest in the use of large flaps of hair-bearing skin taken from the side of the head and turned to cover the balding area (see Fig. 7). As has already been mentioned, there is an essential difference between a graft and a flap. Grafts consist of tissues that are removed *in toto* from their original site and transferred to another. The success or take of a graft containing more than one type of tissue (for example a hair-bearing or full-thickness graft comprising fat, skin and hair follicles) is dictated by the vascularity of the new bed (i.e., the number of blood vessels with which it is supplied) and the size of the graft. Punch grafts, for instance, are particularly successful in that they are small, with a diameter not exceeding 4 mm, and implanted in the richly vascularized bed of the scalp.

A flap, on the other hand, although likewise excised, is left attached to the donor area by means of a pedicle, which continues to supply it with blood and thus ensures the survival of all the tissues, including the hairs. The drawback of this technique is that the pedicle obviously restricts the mobility of the flap and limits its use to an adjacent site, although the distance a flap can be moved does vary and depends on the actual length and basal width of its pedicle. Another disadvantage is that a wound corresponding in length to the flap is left in the donor site, so clearly wound closure, scar formation and subsequent disguise have to be taken into account when considering the desirability of a flap and its length. The risk has also to be borne in mind that, in the rare event of the flap failing, a large area of normal hair-bearing skin will have been

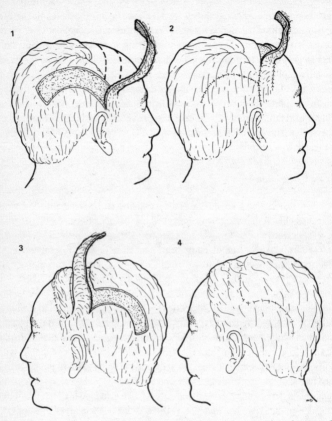

Fig. 7 Hair can also be redistributed by means of one or more hair-bearing flaps moved from the side to the front of the scalp. The wound left in the donor area is closed to form a long scar.

lost from the scalp of a man who is already suffering an unacceptable amount of hair loss.

What a flap does offer to offset these disadvantages, however, is an instant frontal hairline in which all the tissues survive intact and in which any small lacks or defects can easily be made good with the aid of appropriate punch grafts or a well-matched hair-piece. Naturally this technique is a more major undertaking than grafting and may have to be carried out under general anaesthesia, but in any event the patient is usually treated as a day case. The commonest complication of the operation itself is bleeding, and a small drain is inserted and kept in for the first two days to allow blood to escape from the flap where it would otherwise collect and jeopardize its survival. Since only one flap can be transposed at a time, further sessions are required to complete the process, usually at intervals of three months.

Although impressive results have been obtained with flaps, they are not used as frequently as hair-bearing grafts, which remain the mainstay of surgery for baldness.

[11]

Prominent Ears

Children can be unbearably cruel, as every adult knows from experience. Teasing and bullying are an everyday occurrence in childhood, and regardless of the stainless character and flawless looks of a victim, some aspect of his behaviour or appearance will undoubtedly be picked out by classmates and ridiculed. What joy for the bully who finds a child with ears that stick out: an instant nickname of Mr Spock, Batman or Dumbo is bestowed and the child taunted with it thereafter. If sensitive, the child will inevitably suffer, and may even be subject to severe mental stress as a result.

Fortunately, not all children with protruding ears are harmed by teasing. Many have sufficient resilience and character to cope with it, and even the ingenuity to turn their 'handicap' to advantage (indeed, Bing Crosby used to claim that he became famous because of and not in spite of his ears). The implication is that not every child with this potential problem (it can hardly be called a deformity as it is a common variation of the normal) is necessarily a candidate for surgery, particularly since there are also potential psychological dangers for a child undergoing hospitalization and surgical treatment. All the same, parents sometimes find it difficult to accept the doctor's verdict of 'no treatment' when, acting in what they believe to be the best interests of their child, they seek advice, and much more so if they themselves had to endure teasing during childhood for the same reason – which is quite likely, since members of the same family often share protruding ears.

Since there are no means of predicting which child will be teased and suffer most, treatment has to be after the event rather than before, and the child will unfortunately have to run the gauntlet at school. Only when there are overt signs of teasing or, more to the point, when the child itself asks for something to be done, will surgery be considered. This may be a rather crude system of selection for treatment, but at least it avoids a surgeon operating unnecessarily on large numbers of children. It follows from this that surgery is carried out only after the age of six, a procedure further justified by the fact that an ear which may seem unduly prominent up to the age of two or three usually becomes less conspicuous over the next two years as the head grows. Of greater significance is the fact that the ears continue to grow up to the age of six, when they reach near adult proportions, and there is a real hazard that an operation performed before this time will impair normal growth.

While the majority (90 per cent) of patients undergoing surgery for correction of prominent ears are children, 10 per cent consist of young adults who, whether because they become more conscious of their appearance generally or because a new hairstyle attracts undue attention to their ears, also decide in favour of treatment. The prospective patient may equally be a young woman wanting to wear her hair up or a youngster who has entered the Armed Forces and is forced to adopt the short haircut which is a requirement of his new job.

Surgery for Prominent Ears

As Fig. 8 shows, the two main features of a prominent ear are the larger than average bowl or concha and the unusual angle it forms with the side of the head, together with the incompletely developed antihelical fold in the upper third of the ear. These features may occur either separately or in combination.

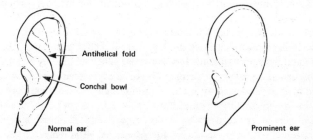

Fig. 8 A prominent ear is characterized by a large conchal bowl set at an angle from the head and/or an incompletely developed antihelical fold. The treatment is to reduce the size of the bowl and scroll the fold more tightly.

The goal of surgery is to reduce the size of the concha and its angle with the head, and to scroll the flattened cartilage in the upper third of the ear to form a new antihelical fold. To this end, an incision is made behind the ear, the skin peeled away from the underlying framework of cartilage, and the latter remodelled and selectively trimmed to the desired shape. The skin is then replaced and the wound closed. As the ear will now lie closer to the head, the scar will be well hidden and will escape notice unless someone actively looks for evidence of surgery (see Fig. 9).

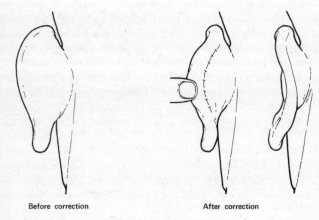

Before correction   After correction

Fig. 9 The scar left after correction lies hidden in the groove at the back of the ear.

Older children and adults should be able to tolerate surgery under local rather than general anaesthesia, injected all round the base of the ear and completely numbing in effect. However, although the operation itself is completely painless, patients may be a little disturbed by a loud scratching noise during sculpting of the cartilage, so young children are usually better off with a general anaesthetic. In either case, the patient is generally discharged on the same day. A heavily padded dressing retained with a head bandage and adhesive tape is worn for the first ten days or so, after which time any sutures are also removed, although as the back of the ear is more than usually sensitive at this stage, sutures which dissolve by themselves are preferred by some surgeons. If, during this period, the dressing becomes too loose or is displaced, as is common in children, a new dressing should immediately be applied. It is certainly unnecessary to keep the child away from school for the ten days when the head bandage is in place, although sporting activities, particularly contact sports such as rugby football and soccer, should be avoided for at least six weeks. Some children may be apprehensive about returning to school wearing a head bandage, but sooner or later their friends will have to know that their ears have been treated, and it might as well be sooner rather than later. However, if parents feel strongly that their child should not go to school with bandages, the operation can be planned to coincide with the school holidays.

Immediately after the dressings have been removed, the ear will be swollen, bruised and tender, and certainly disappointing for anyone expecting an instant improvement. However, as the swelling subsides in the next four weeks the true convolutions of the ear will start to appear. It is a good idea to wear a protective head bandage at night during this period, while the hair, even though it may be washed as normal, should be blow-dried or left to dry naturally, as accidental rubbing of the ears with a towel is painful. Cotton buds (the type used to clean babies' ears and nostrils) soaked in warm water should be used to remove any crusts and debris from the crevices of the ears.

Problems and Complications

An uncomfortable first night after the operation is inevitable, but the pain can usually be countered with the aid of simple analgesic tablets. However, persistent pain over the following days and nights sufficient to interfere with sleep is not normal and is a symptom of infection, excessive bleeding or both. Rather than ignore the signs and continue taking pain-killers, the patient should contact the hospital and return to the ward or out-patients' department so that the dressings can be removed and the underlying cause treated. Infection is rare but is to be avoided at all costs, since if it involves the framework of the ear, part of the cartilage may be destroyed, leaving a permanent deformity.

One of the commonest complications, which arises on the tenth day or thereabouts, is the appearance of a small, shallow ulcer in the frontal area overlying the ridge of the newly constructed antihelical fold. This can occur with the best-insulated dressing and is simply the consequence of pressure transmitted to the ear during sleep, when the patient lies on one side. However, the ulcer usually heals promptly without treatment once the dressing has been removed. Another complication is a haematoma (a collection of blood forming a swelling). This is treated by simple evacuation, and entails neither long-term damage nor risk of a 'cauliflower ear', which is a permanent deformity following repeated small haemorrhaging between the skin and the cartilage over a number of years, such as occurs among rugby forwards and professional boxers.

Treatment of prominent ears is both a safe proposition and one with a happy outcome for the patient, but surgeons are only human and imperfect surgery is always a possibility, as inadequate correction or over-correction of protruding ears sometimes shows. However, over-correction and minor degrees of residual protrusion are often quite acceptable to the patient, and even if any undesirable defects are seen, these will be minor and easily corrected by further surgery, carried out after an interval of at least three months.

[12]

Surgery of the Nose

The demand for rhinoplasty, the repair or modification of the nose, is such as to have made this the leading field in cosmetic surgery. Whatever a patient's motivation for surgery, whether a wish to correct a defect arising from some previous injury or simply dislike for his nose, surgeons who carry out this type of operation (usually plastic surgeons or ear, nose and throat specialists) acknowledge that a rhinoplasty is one of the most testing of all cosmetic procedures – not only because it is technically demanding but also because misunderstandings can so easily arise between the surgeon and the patient as to what the latter wants, especially if due care is not taken in the planning stages, with detailed notes and photographs backing up the discussions. A surgeon can do more than a hundred and one things to change a nose, but all his efforts will be wasted if the final result is not what the patient originally had in mind.

It is helpful if the patient arrives at the interview knowing clearly what features of the nose he dislikes, so that the discussion can quickly focus on what is important – the feasibility of the proposed changes. Most surgeons plan a rhinoplasty with the aid of specially taken pre-operative photographs, but it is even more helpful if the patient brings detailed photographs (consisting of side and front views of the face) that he has studied before the interview, and indicates exactly what is to be changed (although showing pictures of a favourite film star and demanding a nose to match will seldom earn a surgeon's sympathy: the film star's nose may look very well on its owner but is hardly likely to do anything for the patient). Equally, the patient should come to the consultation with an open mind and be prepared to accept alternative suggestions from the surgeon if the latter feels, on the basis of past experience, that what the patient wants is not in his best interests.

The surgeon can easily demonstrate this by marking the patient's suggested changes on a photograph with a felt-tip pen and thus pointing out the problems that are likely to arise. The patient may then realize that the original plan was wrong and agree to modify it. In certain cases, the photograph may even show that it is not the nose that is at fault but an altogether different feature of the face, for example a receding chin.

A consultation may sometimes lead a surgeon to suspect that rhinoplasty, or any other operation for that matter, could be harmful and that psychiatric assessment and treatment would be more appropriate, so he will occasionally refer a patient to a psychiatrist. Anxiety and depression are not uncommon, and the psychiatrist may find serious underlying problems that are best treated without recourse to surgery or that may even be exacerbated by surgery. Equally well, of course, the psychiatrist may conclude that the surgeon's suspicions were quite unfounded and that rhinoplasty is the right treatment after all. Whatever the case, the patient should never take offence at a suggestion to see another doctor, and certainly not jump to the conclusion that what is implied is insanity. The surgeon is simply calling on a specialist to help in a field, human behaviour in this case, in which he has not been trained – as any other responsible doctor will do when faced with a potential problem outside his preserve.

Surgery

Rhinoplasty is not a minor procedure, and all the usual pre-operative preparations in the form of medical examinations, blood tests and interviews regarding previous significant illnesses are a matter of course. In Britain the operation itself is usually performed under general rather than local anaesthesia (not the case in countries such as the USA), and lasts between thirty minutes and one and a half hours. The overall time spent in hospital depends on the extent of the operation and on what the surgeon deems necessary, but the patient can generally expect to be hospitalized for one to three days. It should perhaps be mentioned at this point that surgery before the age of sixteen is not advised as it tends to interfere with normal nasal growth, while after forty the ageing of the overlying skin and the changing character of the nose make the results difficult to predict, so that the optimum time for treatment is in fact between the ages of twenty and thirty.

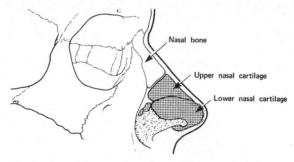

Fig. 10 The structure of the nose depends on the shape, size and position of the nasal bones, cartilages and central septum (the partition between the nostrils), as well as the thickness of the skin and underlying fat.

The basic shape of the nose is determined by the underlying framework of bone and cartilage, the more subtle contours by the disposition and thickness of the tissues in and beneath the skin (see Fig. 10), and it is these components that a surgeon modifies in changing a patient's nose. Most such modifications are carried out via the nostrils, and since the cuts are made in the lining of the nose the resulting scars are virtually undetectable. Even where incisions are made on the outside, care is taken to locate them in the natural groove at the junction of the nose and cheek so that they will not easily be seen. The possibilities for change are many, but basically consist either of augmentation, reduction, or straightening (see Fig. 11).

Reduction rhinoplasty (that is, treatment to reduce the size and prominence of a nose) is by far the commonest nose operation and at its simplest consists of sculpting the cartilages and bones supporting respectively the lower and upper halves of the nose. Complications such as displacement or deviation of the septum (the central partition dividing the nose into two), leading to a twisted nose and sometimes to difficulty in breathing, can be dealt with at the same time, in this case the septum being realigned and the nose made straight, but bone and cartilage manipulation has to be supplemented with thinning of the actual tissues when treatment is for a full, flat nose of the type seen in certain coloured ethnic groups and in the occasional Caucasian. Here, although the thick, soft tissues underlying the skin can be reduced in bulk and other changes successfully implemented to modify the shape of the nose overall (see Fig. 12),

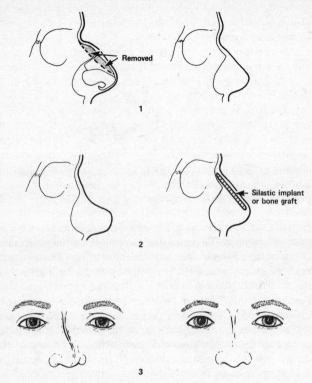

Fig. 11 Rhinoplasty can reduce a large nose (1); augment a 'saddle' nose by means of grafts or a silicone strut (2); and straighten a twisted nose (3).

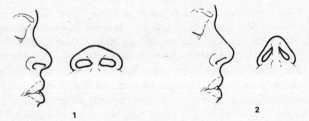

Fig. 12 A flat, full nose (1) can be changed by augmenting and lifting the bridge and tip and by realigning the nostrils (2).

the remodelled tip of a full nose will never have the fine angles and planes of a nose that has undergone cartilage reduction but that is characterized by a thinner layer of skin.

The reverse of this technique is augmentation rhinoplasty, which comes into its own in cases where the bridge has collapsed after disease or injury, for example due to repeated damage in professional boxing, or else when a nose is unduly small or concave. Augmentation is achieved with the aid of bulking or supporting materials implanted in the nose, and here the choice lies between an artificial silicone implant and a bone or cartilage graft taken from the patient's own body. Each of these materials has particular advantages and disadvantages which, together with the nature of the nasal defect and the surgeon's and patient's preferences, are taken into account in any decision as to technique. Grafts taken from the patient's body are particularly advantageous in that there is less likelihood of infection and extrusion than with a foreign material, but a cartilage graft is usually preferable to a bone graft in that little trace is left of the grafting process at the donor site. The required amount of cartilage can be taken either from the ear, via a small cut at the back, or from extraneous cartilage in the nose itself, with no deformation of either structure. If the nasal defect is so pronounced as to render a cartilage graft inadequate, a bone graft taken from a rib or hip-bone has to be used instead, with the inevitable drawback of several days of discomfort and a permanent scar in the donor area. The great advantage of silicone is firstly that there is no question of scars or donor sites and secondly that it is available in any amount and can be carved into any shape whatever. However, since it also entails a marginally higher risk of infection and extrusion, many surgeons prefer not to use it.

After-care and Complications

A broken nose is swollen, tender and bruised, and bleeds under the skin towards the eyelids, causing discoloration and swelling in that area, or into the nostrils as a nose-bleed. A rhinoplasty has exactly the same effects and requires identical treatment in the form of gentle packing of the nostrils with gauze, splinting of the nose with plaster of paris, and cold packs on the eyes. Obviously, until the gauze packs are removed on the second or third day the patient can breathe only through the mouth. For ten days or so he will also feel a strong urge to pick the crusts caking the lining of the nose and partially obstructing the entrance, but should resist the temptation in order to avoid the complication of early, heavy nose-bleeds. If these do occur the usual precaution of sitting with the head thrown back and plugging the nostrils with lint is generally enough to stop the bleeding, but if despite these measures the latter persists, medical aid must be sought. The swelling and bruising round the eyes settle within a week, but there may be residual yellow staining of the lower eyelid skin on removal of the splint after ten to fourteen days, as well as tiny pustules in the skin of the nose. These, together with all plaster marks, can be cleansed with warm water and soap. The hair can at last be washed and it is now safe to blow the nose and clean its lining with cotton buds soaked in plain or salt water. The nose will be delicate for some time, and potentially harmful activities such as contact sports should be avoided for at least three months.

The moment of truth comes when the patient sees the new nose for the first time in the mirror. This can be a less than pleasant experience, for even if the result is exactly as anticipated, barring any swelling which mars the effect, the patient can still find the real thing something of a shock. Such a reaction is entirely natural and the patient must expect an adjustment period of at least a few weeks, if not several months, before he can feel at ease with the stranger in the glass. Moreover, although any obvious swelling will have disappeared after a few weeks, the lower third and tip of the nose will continue to be swollen, if to a less perceptible degree, for six to twelve months, so that the patient will also have to wait a considerable length of time for the finer details to resolve themselves.

Even in the most experienced hands the final result is not always what the patient and surgeon originally had in mind, which, although depressing for both parties, can be so frustrating for the patient in particular that he will sometimes feel impelled to find another surgeon post-haste in order to rectify the fault. The patient is naturally quite entitled to seek a second opinion but should realize that the problem may be seriously compounded if revisional surgery is carried out before the tissues of the nose have settled, i.e., before the end of six months. In fact, unless relationships between the two have become irretrievably soured, it is wiser for the patient to remain under the care of the first surgeon, who after all has first-hand knowledge of his character and nasal anatomy, and who is therefore in the best position to make any minor adjustments that may be necessary to achieve what was planned in the first place.

[13]

The Facial Skeleton

The wars of this and the previous century have been particularly note-worthy in giving surgeons the task of rebuilding shattered faces, but injury and disease take enough of a toll in peacetime for surgeons to have gained considerable everyday experience both in mending broken jaws and other portions of the facial skeleton and in reconstituting the soft tissues over-lying the damaged bones. The lessons learned in the management of such injuries have in the last thirty years been adapted to the benefit of men and women born with facial defects, for the principles at work in the repair and restoration of the face after injury can be applied equally well to the reassembly of bones that have been deliberately fractured by the surgeon for the sake of facial improvement. Just as the shape of a nose can be changed by adjusting its bony and cartilaginous framework, so can the shape of a chin and jaw be altered by sculpting or building up the bone, making a receding chin more prominent or a protruding chin smaller and generally improving the balance of the face. In the last decade the principle has been taken even further in the pioneering work of Paul Tessier, a French surgeon who not only adjusts the upper and lower jaws but also juggles the position of the orbits and the bones of the skull to mend the appearance of children suffering from rare but major congenital malformations of the head and face. However, in the normal course of events, cosmetic surgeons specializing in facial surgery have mainly to deal with problems of the lower jaw, or mandible, and it is to this part of the face that their energies are directed.

The fact that jaws bear teeth and that the upper and lower teeth meet at rest and in chewing is helpful in allowing the surgeon to analyse the relationship between the upper and lower jaws and thus the balance of the face, and the occlusion of the teeth (i.e., the relation between the surfaces when in contact) is in fact the basis for a sound, practical classification of all common jaw deformities. In more sophisticated systems of analysis the surgeon assesses whatever defect is present by plotting various points and angles on a standardized X-ray of the patient's head and measuring the distance between the base of the skull, the nose, the upper and lower jaws and the teeth. The normal range for measurements of this kind has been carefully worked out for the male and female face at different ages and is used as a basis for planning any correction. Although at one time surgeons held that there was such a thing as an ideal face and to prove their theory studied the facial parameters of a group of famous actors and models, they found that the angles and distances varied widely within the group, if fitting into what is considered as the normal range. There is in fact no formula for beauty, and the goal of treating an ugly or rejected facial feature should simply be to modify it in the direction of the 'norm' so that it suits its owner rather than matches its counterpart on the face of some hero or heroine.

Additional aids to planning are plaster models of the teeth and jaws, X-rays, life-size standardized black and white photographs, and three-dimensional working models in the form of plaster moulages or casts of the face. Very recently expensive high technology in the form of computerized axial and three-dimensional tomography has also been introduced, but this is used for gross deformities of the face, upper jaw and skull rather than for the commoner defects of the lower jaw.

It is surprising neither that the leading practitioners in this field of surgery have become oral and maxillo-facial surgeons nor that they have to work closely with other specialists. These include orthodontists (literally 'tooth straighteners'), one of whose skills is cephalometric analysis (measurement of the head and determination of its dimensions and proportions) from which the blueprint for surgery is derived, and technical staff, who cast the actual models and splints, working in a laboratory traditionally associated with an oral surgery department. In Britain, patients requiring corrective jaw surgery are therefore usually managed by a team captained by the oral surgeon and comprising an orthodontist, a dental technician and a plastic surgeon, who may be called upon to perform surgery additional to correction of the jaw-bones themselves, such as revision of the soft-tissue profile or adjustment of the nose, in order to improve the overall balance of the face.

Preparation for Surgery of the Lower Jaw

As every good sculptor knows, detailed plans are essential if a piece is to succeed, and he will use preliminary sketches, drawings, cartoons and models as a matter of course before embarking on the main work. If the sculpture does not meet the artist's standards it will be discarded and started again. A surgeon is not so fortunate: the patient's head cannot be thrown away. Careful preparation is thus even more important than in the sculptor's case and the planning will inevitably take more time and deliberation than the actual execution. Two and sometimes three visits are made to the surgeon over a period of four to six weeks before the date of the operation is definitely fixed.

During the first visit the health in general is assessed and the state of the jaw-bones and teeth in particular examined to check for any disease that might underlie the deformity or put the treatment at risk. Dental impressions are made from which plaster models can be cast, and standardized X-rays taken of the head in such a way as to show the soft-tissue profile and its relation to the facial skeleton. Photographs are taken for planning and records. In the succeeding weeks the oral surgeon and orthodontist analyse the cephalometric values and, aided by X-rays and life-size photographs cut up into segments and juggled into new positions rather in the way an identikit picture of an unknown criminal is built up in front of a witness, decide what should be done in order to improve the patient's face. In the laboratory the jaws and teeth are modelled in plaster and accurately measured for the proposed lengthening, shortening or other adjustment, while the facial profile finally agreed on by the surgeon and orthodontist is built up from their modified X-rays and photographs. During the final visit the operative plan is explained to the patient, any further changes discussed and a date for surgery arranged.

The five deformities of the chin and lower jaw most commonly treated by surgery (normally performed after the age of eighteen, when the facial skeleton is fully developed) are:

1. A small jaw with malocclusion or faulty alignment of the teeth (micrognathia), treated by advancing and lengthening the mandible and enlarging it with the help of a bone graft.
2. A recessed but normal-sized jaw with malocclusion (retrognathia), treated by lengthening the mandible with or without the use of a bone graft.

3. A large, projecting lower jaw with abnormal dental occlusion (prognathism), treated by excising the excess bone and shortening the mandible.

4. A small, recessed chin with normal occlusion of the teeth (microgenia), treated by augmenting the chin alone.

5. A large, prominent chin with normal dental occlusion (macrogenia), effectively treated by trimming the unwanted bone.

Shortening or Lengthening the Lower Jaw

The day before surgery, individually designed splints are fixed to the upper and lower teeth, for reasons that will become apparent later. On the day of the operation, after all the usual preparations for general anaesthesia and pre-operative procedures, incisions are made within the mouth, thus giving access to the mandible, which is then cut with a high-speed air drill along pre-planned lines. If the mandible is to be lengthened, stepped cuts are made in the bone, thereby dividing it into two pieces which are then moved apart the appropriate distance before being fixed in the new position with wires or screws. The technique is very similar to that used in a carpenter's lapped joint. Alternatively, and more commonly, the jaw-bone is divided by an oblique cut rather like that in a scarf joint, which as before allows the two segments to slide apart into their new positions. The two types of joint are illustrated in Fig. 13. If the mandible is so recessed as to require significant extension, bone grafts taken from the hip-bone may be necessary to fill out the gaps between the two segments and stabilize the jaw, the grafting process as usual entailing a scar in the donor area and causing temporary pain in walking.

Once the desired length has been achieved the dental apparatus on the upper jaw will exactly meet and match that on the lower jaw. The mandibular fragments can now be screwed together and the wound

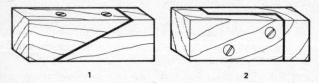

Fig. 13 The jaw-bone is usually fixed by a technique similar to that in a carpenter's scarf joint (1), but a lapped joint can also be used (2).

in the mouth closed before locking together the upper and lower teeth with wires and stout elastic bands passed round the orthodontic splints.

The commoner deformity of an over-large jaw is treated using the same oblique cut but with the obvious difference of telescopic shortening of the two fragments, which then overlap into a scarf joint. Excess bone may have to be removed at the same time.

The patient's appearance immediately after either form of surgery is similar to that of an individual treated for a fractured jaw or with the back molar teeth removed, the face being swollen to the extent where the patient resembles a hamster with full cheek pouches. The first two days are uncomfortable but made as tolerable as possible with the help of pain-killers. Antibiotics, started the day before surgery, are continued for a week to reduce the chance of infection in the sites where the bones were cut. Nevertheless the patient can get out of bed on the first day and can usually go home after five days. The facial swelling will rapidly subside so that by the end of the week there will be little to show for the surgical trauma, and the patient will be able to start work after a fortnight.

The main handicap with which the patient must live for the six to eight weeks until the bones have mended is the immobilization of the upper and lower jaws. Normal speech is possible with the teeth fixed together, as lip mobility is unimpaired, but it is certainly impossible to eat normal meals and all nourishment has to be taken in fluid form. The patient may as a result lose weight during this time (one of the more drastic ways of making people diet is in fact to wire their teeth together), which can be an added bonus for the overweight but a disadvantage where not desired. Weight loss is by no means a foregone conclusion, however, and it is possible not only to maintain weight with a liquid diet but actually to put it on. What should perhaps be stressed is that the occasional patient can experience such a frightening feeling of suffocation as a result of his jaws being wired together that anyone undergoing this form of treatment is advised to carry a pair of scissors or wire-cutters in case of emergency. However, the retaining wires or bands should be cut only as a last resort.

Complications

It must be understood that cosmetic surgery to lengthen or shorten the lower jaw is quite feasible but that it is a major operation and complications can therefore arise.

A single large nerve serves the lower teeth, the sides of the tongue, the chin and all the mandible as far as the back teeth and slightly beyond, passing through bone and soft tissue in the process. Injury of any part of this nerve affects the whole area, and it is for this reason that a dentist injecting local anaesthetic around the lower teeth prior to drilling and filling incidentally numbs the tongue and chin as well. The surgeon therefore takes great pains to identify, preserve and protect the nerve during the splitting and mobilization of the jaw-bones but even so may occasionally stretch or injure it, leaving the lips, teeth and chin completely numb for up to three months, the time required for the nerve to heal.

Excessive bleeding, a rare complication, is treated with the aid of compressive dressings and bandages, while infection, likewise uncommon, is treated simply by drainage and administration of antibiotics.

Occasionally the rebuilt mandible fails to consolidate into its new shape, giving rise to painful instability of the jaw and making speaking and eating difficult. The problem may be solved by having the patient wear the orthodontic apparatus and link wires for a further six weeks, or, should this measure fail, by inserting a bone graft into the freshened lining of the fracture site in combination with further immobilization of the teeth. Minor degrees of relapse towards the original deformity may be acceptable, depending on the patient, but if not the surgeon will perform corrective surgery, the only adequate measure in this case.

Enlarging or Reducing the Chin

In contrast to surgery for the lower jaw, surgery on the chin alone is relatively safe and simple, allowing a short stay in hospital and an early return to work. Moreover, since in this case the under-development or over-development of the bony prominence on the lower jaw is uncomplicated by faulty alignment of the teeth, planning of the correction, based on photographs of the face and X-rays of the chin, is much less elaborate and difficult than for an abnormally long or small lower jaw as a whole.

Chin Reduction

Where the chin is to be reduced, the soft tissues covering the bone of the chin are peeled away via a horizontal cut made in the gutter between the lower lip and the lower front teeth (or in some cases via a small

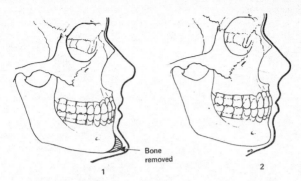

Bone
removed

1   2

Fig. 14 A large chin on a normally positioned jaw is treated simply by chiselling or drilling away the excess bone (1). A better profile is thus obtained (2).

skin incision on the undersurface of the chin, the sutures used to close the wound being removed about a week later) and the excess bone removed with an air drill, a small power-driven reciprocating saw or a hammer and chisel. The tissues are then sutured back into place (see Fig. 14). The operation can be performed under local anaesthesia but, in view of the noise accompanying the carpentry, most surgeons prefer to use a general anaesthetic and so avoid causing distress.

The patient can leave hospital the next day but has to observe certain precautions, such as keeping to a soft diet for the first three to five days and taking a course of antibiotics, usually prescribed for a week. Any local tenderness, swelling and bruising will have settled within a few days, when male patients can comfortably shave once more, and work can usually be resumed after a week. A specific and not infrequent complication is minor injury to the sensory nerve as it emerges from the bone into the skin of the chin with ensuing numbness. This however lasts only a few months, as long, in fact, as it takes for the nerve to recover.

A particularly large chin cannot adequately be reduced by simple excision of the excess bone and must be remodelled by rearranging a segment of the bone and wiring it into the new position. Since local reaction is correspondingly great, the patient may need to remain in hospital for a further day and to stay away from work for a fortnight.

Chin Augmentation

A cosmetic surgeon is generally reluctant to comment on a patient's physiognomy and to suggest improvements, and leaves the patient to pinpoint any problems before discussing the possibilities of correction. An exception to the rule is, however, sometimes made in the case of chin augmentation, a possibility that seldom even occurs to the patient but which is useful in achieving a better overall balance of the face and thus a more pleasing appearance. For a surgeon to suggest such an operation and therefore to imply an additional defect (chin augmentation is usually proposed in connection with nasal reduction: 5 per cent of all patients undergoing rhinoplasty in the USA, 2 per cent in Britain, are also given a chin implant) may seem impertinent, but experience in the USA has shown that patients are usually quite happy with the surgeon's proposal and are virtually always satisfied with the result.

The chin can be enlarged either by means of a silicone implant (see Fig. 15) or by sliding forward a wedge of bone and wiring it into place, the choice of technique depending on the size and shape of the chin. The incisions, post-operative aspects, after-care and complications are similar to those associated with chin reduction.

The silicone chin prosthesis has the advantage of being easily implanted under local anaesthesia with the patient as a day case, unless associated with a rhinoplasty, but can be complicated in the longer term with

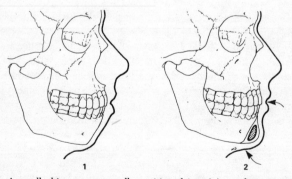

Fig. 15 A small chin on a normally positioned jaw (1) can be augmented by means of a silicone implant inserted via an incision either inside the mouth or in the skin of the upper neck (2).

untoward shifting of the implant, infection and extrusion. A slipped prosthesis is a simple matter of surgical repositioning, but if infection sets in, as rarely happens, the implant must be removed, and replaced only after an interval of at least three months. Sculpting a very small chin is a bigger job, requiring general anaesthesia and the same after-care as with segmental remodelling of the very large chin.

Remodelling the Cheeks

The high cheek-bones requested by some patients can be achieved by inserting custom-designed silicone implants into pockets cut out from the skin over the cheek-bones and approached either by a cut made just in front of the ear or an incision high inside the mouth. The result can be dramatically effective but the surgery has risks and hazards identical to those of any comparable operation involving silicone.

A few individuals acquire powerful cheek muscles which make them unusually, and sometimes unacceptably, square of face. The cause of these is unknown but unrelated to excessive use: they are as likely to occur in a petite vegetarian as in a steak-eating lumberjack. The muscle can be reduced in size by trimming away the inner fibres via a cut under the angle of the jaw or within the mouth, but there is a potential complication of injury to the facial nerve animating the face, and a temporary facial weakness is occasionally seen.

[14]

Facelift and Chemical Peel

Judging by the plethora of articles and advertisements in the average women's journal and by the flood of books on the subject, rejuvenation appears to be the middle-aged female's chief preoccupation; indeed, it is difficult to turn a page without encountering a lotion, cream, unguent, skin preparation or treatment that does not hold out the promise of new life for the tired face (faces are always tired, never old). To the facial massage, hot pack, cold pack and mud pack of the beauty parlour, high technology has now added laser therapy, which claims, despite an absolute paucity of scientific evidence, to achieve the same goals as a facelift – miraculously, it would seem. It is obvious, of course, that it is neither a universal nor an entirely female obsession to check or reverse the flow of time, that no cream or mud pack can wipe out or ward off the effects of age, that facelifts provide only a semblance – temporary, at that – of youth, and that there are no miracles. Yet there are many who ontinue to believe in magic solutions. Whatever the case, knowing something about the composition of the soft tissues of the face will help prospective patients understand what a facelift can and cannot achieve (see also Chapter 3, 'The Ageing of Skin').

The soft tissues overlying the bony framework of the face and neck are made up of three layers, each susceptible to the effects of age. The deepest consists of a complex arrangement of muscles which, by virtue of their contracting power, allow movement of the face and neck and thus intricate variations of facial expression. The thin, large sheet of muscle known as the platysma, suspended from the jaw and extending into the neck, functions as a support for the neck (essentially like a built-in chin strap), giving the younger person a taut, flat chin and a well-defined angle at the junction of the neck and jaw. As this muscle ages and loses its tone, however, gravity takes its toll and pulls the flesh out of shape, making it bulge downwards in the form of a jowl and blurring the normal angle between the neck and jaw. Further loss of tone leads to vertical ridges of muscle which, overhung by slackened skin, produce marked folds in the neck – a process sometimes referred to rather unkindly as the turkey-gobbler effect. The topmost layer consists of the skin. Here, creaselines are a normal feature even in youth and can be seen in a crying baby or a laughing child, but are smoothed away as soon as the face comes to rest and the young elastic tissue in the skin springs back into place. In the process of ageing, however, which is accelerated by prolonged exposure to sunlight, the skin gradually loses its elasticity, and the creaselines become fixed in the form of grooves or wrinkles in areas of greatest mobility, for example around the eyes, mouth and forehead (less mobile areas such as the upper cheek do not acquire permanent wrinkles until much later in life). The third layer, sandwiched between the muscle and the skin, is made up of fat. Although in youth this is uniformly distributed over the central and lower thirds of the face, in later years and under the effect of gravity it tends to shift downwards into the neck and jaw, emphasizing the jowl and progressively increasing the hollow of the cheeks.

Excision of redundant facial skin may thus not always be enough to solve the problem of sagging folds and wrinkles, and to achieve the full effect a facelift will probably also need to include partial excision and remodelling of the fat in the neck and lower part of the face and trimming and tightening of the platysma. It may now be appreciated that a full facelift is a major operation lasting between $2\frac{1}{2}$ and $3\frac{1}{2}$ hours and that patients must be in good general health to be accepted for surgery.

Facelifts

The average age for a facelift is fifty-five, the optimum time for surgery lying between the ages of forty-five and sixty-five. Although facelifts in men are increasingly in demand (2 per cent of all patients undergoing surgery in the United Kingdom and 10 per cent in the USA are male), the results are not as good as in women, since male facial skin is bearded and thicker and predisposed to a slightly higher risk of complications. A full, fat face, whether it be male or female, is very difficult to treat effectively, and an overweight patient is usually advised against surgery if sufficient weight loss cannot be achieved. The ideal candidate is in fact a slim woman in her late forties or early fifties who reasonably objects to the signs of ageing on her face, who wants to look better for her own and no one else's sake, and who fully realizes the limitations of the operation. A patient who goes into surgery believing that a facelift holds the key to happiness, youth and instant success is hardly likely to benefit in any real sense from the operation.

Patients serious about a facelift should not give much consideration to what is described as a 'mini-lift', since this entails no more than minimal elevation and excision of facial skin, with no improvement of the platysmal neck muscle or redistribution of facial fat. A mini-lift gives a mini-result, and even if a gratifying result is initially obtained as a result of temporary flattening of the creases by post-operative swelling, this will last a matter of months rather than years. Even the full, properly executed facelift has little effect on the forehead or the area around the eyes, which are best treated directly by browlift and eyelid reduction (see Chapter 15), or on the heavy folds between the side of the nose and the angle of the mouth (nasolabial folds). The most dramatic improvement is on the tissues of the neck and lower jaw, the surgeon aiming to give a smooth, clean, naturally curving jawline, to eliminate hanging folds of skin and muscle together with excessive fat beneath the jaw, and to accentuate the normal angle between the neck and the jaw. A facelift is therefore something of a misnomer as the main efforts of the surgeon are directed to the neck and lower third of the face (see Fig. 16).

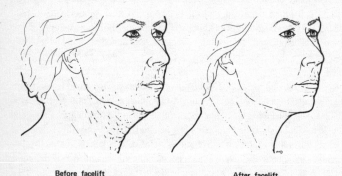

Before facelift   **After facelift**

Fig. 16 The essential goals of a facelift are to improve the lower third of the face overall, to give a cleaner jawline and to provide the neck and underside of the chin with a smoother contour.

The Operation and After-care

In Britain the patient is usually given a general anaesthetic, although there is a growing tendency, as in all cosmetic surgery, to follow the trend set by surgeons in the USA and in certain cases to perform facelifts under local anaesthesia and sedation. Whatever the anaesthetic used the surgical technique remains the same.

The incision for a facelift starts in the hair-bearing area above the ear, continues down to follow the natural crease between the face and the front of the ear, turns round the earlobe and runs round the back of the ear in the groove between the ear cartilage and the bone of the skull up to the thinner and more delicate skin at the hairline behind the ear, before finally veering off at right angles into the hair low on the side of the head (see Fig. 17). A scar along this track is obviously inevitable, but as four fifths

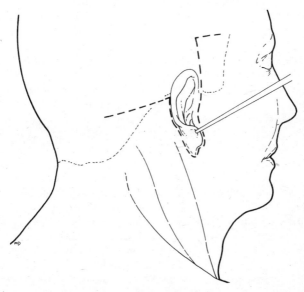

Fig. 17 A typical facelift incision cannot easily be seen: most of it lies either in the hair-bearing area or behind the ear, and what remains runs along the natural crease between the cheek and the front of the ear.

of its length lie either in hair-bearing skin or in the area immediately behind the ear, it remains well hidden. Only the portion in front of the ear and within the creaseline is liable to detection on closer scrutiny.

The facial and neck skin is undermined both to allow an effective skin lift and also to give the surgeon access to fat lying over the platysmal muscle, along the line of the jaw and beneath it. Any excess can thus be trimmed away to leave a more easily visualized muscle sheet, which is then freed at its outer margin and lifted upwards and outwards to be anchored to the edge and surface of the larger neck muscles. Any redundant tissue in the platysma itself can be excised or plicated with the aim of tightening it and therefore providing better support and a smoother contour. The undermined skin can now be lifted in the classical fashion upwards and backwards before being trimmed of excess and fixed in place with sutures. Most of the strain and tension of the skin lift is taken up by the suture line running into the scalp hair behind the ear, which means that sturdier suture materials are needed here than in front of the ear, where the skin lies more comfortably and can therefore be sutured more finely to give a finer scar in the long term. After the main surgery, two tubes, passed through a small hole in the hairline of the neck and connected, under negative pressure, to a small container, are usually inserted under the skin on either side of the face in order to drain off any blood and serum which would otherwise collect. These remain in place for not more than forty-eight hours, after which they are removed together with the encircling head and neck bandages. The puncture sites heal quickly without the need for sutures, leaving a tiny mark easily concealed in the hair.

The first glimpse the patient has of herself in the mirror may be quite startling, for gazing back will be not just a different, slightly swollen face but one almost adolescent in appearance and from which all the main creases will have vanished. Unfortunately, this smooth, youthful face is entirely the effect of post-operative swelling and gradually recovers its original creases, although these will be a little flatter than before. The effect of gravity is useful in reducing the swelling; the patient should try to sit up as much as possible during the day and to lie propped up by as many pillows as possible during the night. She should likewise try to avoid lying on her side in the first seven to ten days in order to prevent one side of her face from swelling more than the other.

A common worry is that the surgeon will shave part of the head before cutting into the hairline and thus leave an extensive bald area. There is no need for anxiety, however, since hair is not a major source of infection in surgery of the face and scalp and is left intact. The only possible irritation as far as the patient is concerned is that the hair will be dirty for some time, since the surgeon is unable to clean the hair adequately at the end of the operation and inevitably leaves it matted both with dry crusts and also with the preparation used for pre-operative cleansing. As soon as the bandages and drains have been removed, however, the hair can be washed and gently blow-dried. At this point the patient can leave hospital and resume her normal life at home, covering the evidence of surgery with a loose headscarf and dark glasses, if necessary, until the stitches have been removed after seven to ten days (the stitches in front of the ear can be taken out a few days earlier). Most patients are not keen to display themselves at this stage and stay quietly at home or with close friends, or even combine the treatment with a holiday. Despite the use of drains and careful sealing and securing of bleeding points at the time of surgery there is a small amount of bruising, spreading to the neck and going through all the usual colour changes of purple to yellow before finally disappearing. The discoloration will usually have gone by the end of two weeks but in any case can easily be disguised by wearing a high collar or a polo-neck or by using light make-up. Patients are advised to take not less than two weeks off from work – not just to allow the face to recover but also to regain sufficient strength and stamina to return to normal life and duties. A facelift is a long and major operation and patients are often surprised at how easily tired they get in the first few weeks after surgery.

Patients are sometimes anxious about facing friends or colleagues for the first time. However, the typical reaction of people unaware of the real reason for their absence is nothing more than surprise at how well they look, the improvement – particularly as it is a subtle change in certain features rather than a dramatic reversal of time – being ascribed to a good holiday or a diet. Remarks such as, 'My God! You've had a facelift!' are extremely unlikely.

As has already been mentioned, improvements of this kind are difficult to achieve in a man. The facial skin is thicker and more difficult to mobilize and rearrange; the scars are less easy to disguise, especially in the case of a thinning and balding scalp; and bearded skin is pulled close to the front of the ear and just behind the earlobe. These drawbacks, as well as the general aspects of a facelift, are explained in detail before surgery, and although they may discourage the occasional patient, the genuinely motivated male can overcome some of the difficulties by shaving behind the ear and a little closer to the front of it and, if necessary, by growing sideburns to cover the scar completely.

How long does a facelift last? Each patient is unique in terms of facial structure, skin thickness and elasticity, degree of ageing, motivation and psychological make-up, and each responds differently to the operation. It is therefore impossible to give an accurate, reliable answer, and surgeons usually find themselves replying in rather vague terms that the degree of success and life of a facelift depend on several factors, that the ageing process has not been reversed or halted, that the rate of ageing varies according to the person and that if, after a few years, there are any unacceptable changes a second facelift can be considered. Unlike a garage mechanic who is able to guarantee a reconditioned engine or a rust-proofed car body, the surgeon cannot give the patient an absolute assurance as to success or durability – and will in any case be particularly reluctant to do so as this will make him vulnerable to litigation.

Complications and Limitations

Regardless of meticulous surgery and securing of bleeding vessels, blood still occasionally leaks into the space beneath the undermined facial skin to form a clot (or haematoma), producing excessive and painful facial swelling. A large haematoma needs to be evacuated as soon as possible. If it does not prove amenable to 'milking' through the suture line in front of or behind the ear or if the haematoma re-forms, the surgeon will have no choice but to give another anaesthetic and re-explore the face to clean out all clots and hunt for any bleeding points. While major haematomas occur only in 2 to 3 per cent of all patients, smaller collections of blood are a little more common, but these can usually be successfully treated without recourse to the operating theatre. If untreated, minor haematomas leave a small thickening in the face which gradually softens and flattens over the next two to four months as the blood is slowly absorbed.

The commonest complication is the death of a small triangle of skin high behind the ear where it is thin and delicate and under maximum tension. Nature is best in treating this problem as the natural sequence of events is for new skin to grow beneath the scab, or eschar, which eventually falls off. Very rarely the skin loss extends below the ear to the neck and even the face. Here, although obviously distressing for the patient, it is once again better to allow nature to run its course without interference, since the long-term results are very satisfactory and infinitely better than those achieved by means of early surgical treatment with a skin graft.

Areas of partial skin death along the scalp incision will also heal spontaneously but the new skin will initially be hairless, since the hair follicles it carries, which behave exactly like those in a punch hair graft (see Chapter 10), start to generate hair only after about six months. The resulting scar will nevertheless be more conspicuous after maturation than those which have healed uneventfully, although since it lies behind the ear and in a hair-bearing area it will generally escape notice.

Two types of nerve can be injured during a facelift: nerves controlling facial animation (motor nerves) and nerves receiving sensation from the face (sensory nerves). In every facelift small, terminal sensory nerves in the undermined skin are inevitably severed during the operation, leaving numb a narrow belt of skin just in front of the incision. Normal sensation does eventually return once these small nerves have healed, but the process may take up to nine or even twelve months. The return of feeling is sometimes accompanied by an aggravating tingling sensation that has been likened to the crawling of ants on the face (hence the word 'formication' to describe it) but which is actually a healthy sign. A large, sensory nerve passing up the side of the neck is also at risk and is injured in 3 per cent of facelifts, rendering the lower half of the ear totally numb. Depending on the degree of injury the nerve may eventually recover, but if not the sensory loss will be permanent. Of greater importance is damage to one of the motor nerve branches (occurring in 1 to 2 per cent of patients) leading to asymmetrical movement of the mouth or forehead. The usual cause is bruising of a nerve during surgery, but in this case recovery is assured (taking from three months to a year) since the nerve has not actually been severed.

Pain or discomfort in the early days after a facelift is commonly associated with a large clot and is relieved as soon as the latter is evacuated, but it also occurs after the sutures have been removed, when patients often experience a tight, uncomfortable feeling across the neck exacerbated by turning the head from side to side. This discomfort, an effect of hitching up the platysmal muscle to improve the contour of the neck, disappears however once the muscle has stretched.

Where there is a rich blood supply infection is unlikely, and since, with the exception of the attenuated skin behind the ear, the face and scalp are well endowed with healthy blood vessels they are at little risk. If any eschar behind the ear does become infected, however, treatment is easy: the scab is simply removed. Anaesthesia is not required in this case as the fine sensory nerves in that particular area will have been severed during the facelift and will therefore not be functioning.

Occasionally the earlobe becomes slightly distorted and displaced due to contracture of the surrounding scar, but correction is not a problem and is carried out under local anaesthesia.

An after-effect that is not often anticipated is a feeling of regret which may border on depression in the first few days after surgery and particularly while the face is swollen and bruised. This type of reaction is certainly not helped by the relative inactivity and fatigue associated with recovery from major surgery. As after any cosmetic operation and before the results of the treatment have become apparent, patients are likely to ask themselves if the experience has been worthwhile or even justifiable. All the surgeon can do is reassure them that after the bruising and swelling have subsided they will feel much better. In fact it is remarkable how quickly patients return to normal and forget their depression once they have seen the effects of the facelift – providing, of course, that their expectations have not been unrealistic.

By now it will be obvious that the term 'facelift' is somewhat inaccurate, for the predominant effect of the operation is on the neck and jawline alone. The forehead and surrounds of the eyes themselves can be improved only by browlift and blepharoplasty, both of which are discussed in the next chapter. 'Rhytidectomy' is also a misleading term, for the deep creases in the face are not removed but only flattened out to a certain extent. In fact the fine lines and grooves around the mouth and eyes can be effectively treated only by dermabrasion (see Chapter 6) or, better, by chemical peeling, referred to by some surgeons as chemabrasion.

Chemical Face Peel

As its name implies, the technique of chemical face peel makes use of a strong chemical (phenol, mixed in a well-tried and established formula with distilled water, liquid soap and croton oil) to destroy, in effect burn off, the outer layer of the skin and so lay bare a deep layer from which new skin can grow. A full and effective peel cannot be achieved without pain, discomfort and inconvenience, or without the patient looking fairly horrific for a few days. However, by the time the new skin has matured, the finer lines will have disappeared and even the deeper grooves will have become less obvious. The ideal patient is fair-skinned, with minimal skin redundancy and multiple fine wrinkles of the type acquired through prolonged exposure to sunlight over many years.

The face is normally peeled without full anaesthesia, but should any patient be particularly apprehensive a general anaesthetic can be used. The first step is to clean the skin of all make-up and oils and lightly and evenly smear it with a cotton bud soaked in the caustic mixture until the whole surface has turned white. This process is accompanied by a stinging pain, which however disappears in a matter of seconds and can in any case be dampened by appropriate drugs. Once all the relevant surfaces have been treated they are sealed with several layers of adhesive tape, after which the patient returns to bed to rest for two days. During this time the soft tissues around the eyes and mouth swell dramatically: the eyelids close and eating and speaking become difficult, so that the patient may have to communicate with paper and pencil and take fluid through a straw. On the third day the tapes, carrying on their undersurface much of the dead outer layer of skin, are removed, leaving an exquisitely tender, raw surface which is then dusted with an antiseptic powder to form a caked crust. Naturally the removal of the tapes is painful and the patient receives strong pain-killers. From now on the swelling settles, the eyelids open and eating and speaking become less of a problem. On the fifth or sixth day the crust is softened with cold cream or vaseline and gently and relatively painlessly removed with the aid of soap and lukewarm water. The newly formed skin, like that seen after an acute sunburn, will be bright pink and abnormally sensitive to normal stimuli, and unless kept moist with standard face creams and oils will dry and crack. Two weeks after the peel the patient can start to wear light make-up to disguise the now paler discoloration, which will persist for one to three months before completely disappearing.

The complications and disadvantages of a chemical peel are much the same as those associated with a partial-thickness burn. A minor risk is that, if an area is burnt too deeply, the skin will heal by scarring and possibly cause distortion of adjacent structures such as the eyelids or lips. Treatment in this case is along the lines outlined in the chapter on scars. More commonly, multiple tiny white spots appear after two to three weeks, signifying blockage of the sebaceous glands; these are cleared by lightly rubbing the affected area with a soft brush dipped in soap and water. The new skin, which is abnormally sensitive to sunlight and should be protected with creams containing an ultraviolet screen, matures to a colour paler than that of unpeeled skin, which is not necessarily a great problem in a total face peel but can be disadvantageous if only the skin around the eyes and mouth is treated, since the patient ends up looking like a panda. While make-up can in certain cases be quite effective in disguising the bleached area, patients with dark skin are not advised to undergo this form of treatment. In fact the lighter the patient's colouring the better. For obvious reasons a full peel is not performed at the same time as a facelift, but several months later. The risk of complications is higher in other areas, and chemical peel is seldom recommended for sites such as the hands or arms.

Less Common Procedures

In some cases the neck is burdened with so much fat and festooned with so many folds of platysmal muscle that a traditional facelift is not enough. Instead, a horizontal incision is made directly in the natural creaseline below the chin, giving the surgeon easy access to the redundant tissue (see Fig. 18). Once the fat has been sculpted and the muscle trimmed and adjusted, the excess skin is excised and the margins of the wound brought together and sutured.

It has been mentioned that the heavy nasolabial fold of skin and fat stretching from the base of the nose to the corner of the mouth is not something that a facelift can really improve, and the only way to deal with

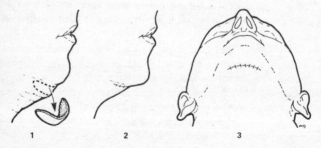

Fig. 18 A conventional facelift cannot cope with excessive amounts of skin and fat in the neck, and the redundant tissue (1) is removed via an incision on the underside of the chin (2, 3).

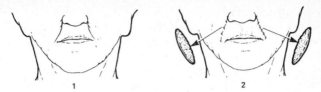

Fig. 19 Heavy folds in the nasolabial area (1) are excised via a cut along the natural creaseline running from the nose to the mouth (2).

it effectively is to cut away the excess tissue. A long scar is inevitable, but fortunately the nasolabial groove hides it reasonably well (see Fig. 19).

An uncommon request is for the surgeon to introduce a facial dimple or to emphasize one that is already there. A cheek dimple is made by cutting through the mucous membrane lining the inside of the mouth, taking out a cone of fat and pulling the skin inwards by means of sutures passed through its deep layer. A chin dimple is produced in much the same way but via a small cut made directly over the point of the chin.

[15]

Correction of the Eyelids
and Upper Face

However unfairly, character is often judged by appearance and conclusions instantly drawn from dress, hairstyle and physiognomy. In that they focus the onlooker's attention, the eyes and the area immediately around them are particularly important in establishing a first impression: for example, lines and folds around and on the eyelids often give an impression of chronic fatigue and age, while puffy eyelids sometimes indicate habitual dissipation and heavy lids a lazy or sleepy nature. The eyebrows and forehead add to the initial impact: drooping, sloping eyebrows convey not only tiredness but sadness, and if combined with deep horizontal furrowing of the forehead create an image of agitation and anxiety. Vertical grooves between the eyebrows, on the other hand, may imply bad temper. All these signs, particularly if misleading and out of character, may be strongly resented by their owners, sometimes to the extent where they will actually want to change them. Here again cosmetic surgery can help.

While a few years ago it was usual for a surgeon to operate selectively on the eyelids, eyebrows or forehead, there is now a growing tendency to adjust all three parts together in order to achieve the right balance.

Baggy Eyelids

Correction of baggy eyelids (blepharoplasty is the technical term for surgery of the eyelids) is, with rhinoplasty, one of the two commonest cosmetic operations on the face, and it is interesting how dramatically the overall appearance of the face can be changed by relatively minor alterations in this area (see Fig. 20). Before any form of surgery is considered, however, it is essential to determine if the puffiness around the eyes has any abnormal cause, since systemic disorders such as certain forms of

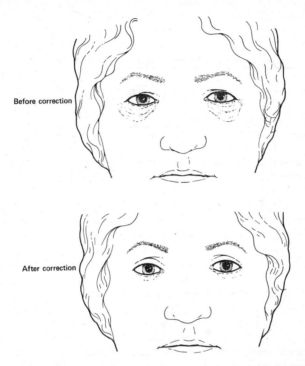

Fig. 20 Upper and lower eyelid correction reduces excess skin, fat and muscle, either singly or in combination. The position of the eyebrows remains unchanged.

kidney or heart disease or hormonal imbalance can be reflected in changes in the eyelid skin. The patient should therefore consult a reputable surgeon who can recognize such phenomena and prescribe treatment through a physician if the need arises. All the same it is very rare for the above disorders to be noticed only as a result of an unusual process in the eyelids, so that not all patients with puffy eyes need worry that they have some dire medical condition. Nevertheless the possibility of an underlying complication should deter them from visiting an inadequately trained surgeon.

Three elements – skin, fat and muscle – can be reduced by blepharo-plasty, either singly or in combination, the amount of tissue excised depending on the individual's needs and on which condition is present. For example, as the skin ages, it can develop an excess of drooping folds in the upper eyelid and creases in the lower eyelid; the loose fat surround-ing and protecting the eyeball can accumulate to an unusual extent, particularly under the lower eyelid, and bulge out under the skin (surplus eyelid fat is frequently a family trait, and appears at a relatively early age); or the ring of muscle encircling the eye and used to screw up the eyes against bright sunlight or by short-sighted people in an effort to see more clearly can become unnaturally bulky when over-used. Each of these conditions requires a slightly different approach.

The Operation

During the examination and interview prior to the operation, which is performed under general or local anaesthesia, the surgeon determines what is at fault and what can be corrected.

Upper eyelid reduction is a relatively quick and troublefree operation, and consists simply of excising the desired amount of skin together with any excess fat and closing the wound with fine sutures. Because the skin in the upper eyelid is extremely delicate and thin, the resulting scar is one of the finest that can be achieved. Moreover, since it lies within a normal skin fold and ends in the natural creases at the outer corner of the eye, it is one of the very few that can be described as truly imperceptible.

The patient can usually return home on the same day, wearing suppor-tive adhesive tapes removed after three to four days, at the same time as the sutures. Any complications relate to excessive bruising and swelling, but these can be overcome by sleeping in a more upright position and using cold compresses on the eyes. Dark glasses can be worn to disguise any residual discoloration, and work and normal duties resumed after a fortnight.

Unlike surgery of the upper eyelid, that of the lower is one of the most exacting cosmetic procedures, fully matching rhinoplasty in its challenge. Unfortunately, as operations become more technically demanding, so the risks and complications mount up, and since reduction of the lower eyelid is no exception the patient is warned of the potential early and late hazards in the initial stages of discussion.

A horizontal cut is made just below the roots of the eyelashes (which are therefore not at risk), extending outwards into the crowsfoot. The skin is pulled downwards to expose the muscle and fat, which are excised and trimmed as necessary. To enable the surgeon to judge how much skin should be removed, the conscious patient is asked to open the eyes and mouth. If, however, a general anaesthetic is being used, this is done by an assistant. Wound closure and post-operative management are exactly the same as for the upper eyelid.

It is now less usual for complete, occlusive eye pads to be used after surgery as already apprehensive patients can become even more agitated at the thought of being completely dependent on others during the post-operative phase. Instead, cold packs are applied intermittently to relieve local discomfort and suppress bruising and swelling.

Complications

Until the sutures and overlying tapes are removed, local swelling can drag the lower eyelid away from contact with the eyeball. In the majority of cases this effect lasts only a week, but during this time the tears usually drained off via the narrow, capillary-like channel at the inner corner of the eye, pool instead in the gutter between the lid and the eye and spill over the edge on to the cheek. At night the undrained tears evaporate to leave the eyelids gummed up with sticky crusts, which have to be cleaned off every morning with a simple eye-wash and cotton buds. As soon as the lower eyelid returns to its normal position, however, the normal drainage mechanism begins to function again and the eyelids become less sticky. If the eyes continue to feel gritty and irritated after the crusts have been removed it is possible that other foreign bodies are present, in which case the patient may be referred to another specialist for investigation and possible treatment.

In addition, the thin membrane covering the eyeball retains water after the operation and becomes glistening and jelly-like, often causing the patient more concern than the excessive watering. Here again, however, the effect wears off within a week.

After seven to ten days, make-up can be gently applied around the eyes to disguise any residual bruising. Sweeping movements with the finger from the top of the nose along the eyelids to the outer corner of the eye not only position the make-up but also help to disperse whatever swelling remains.

A complication that emerges somewhat later is pronounced asymmetry of the two sets of eyelids. Some degree of asymmetry is normal, but if as a result of surgery the eyelids have become obviously unequal, too much or too little fat, skin or muscle having been removed from one eyelid, minor adjustments under local anaesthesia can easily be performed to achieve the right balance.

The most frequent late complication, however, is a longer-standing downward pull on the lower eyelid with an effect ranging from mere exposure of the white of the eye between the lower edge of the iris and the margin of the eyelid, to complete eversion of the latter with all its red lining disclosed. As every surgeon has to admit, the reason for this is the removal of too much skin, and in the event of extreme, permanent lower eyelid eversion the only remedy is a full-thickness skin graft. Smaller degrees of eversion can, however, correct themselves in time as the eyelid skin softens and stretches, while some patients actually find the wide-eyed look acquired through minor eversion quite attractive. Whatever the extent of the complication the eye feels vulnerable, and patients generally feel safer and more comfortable if they wear dark glasses as a protection against sun and wind.

A sunken, hollow-eyed look stems from the removal of too much fat, a loss that fat grafts cannot unfortunately make good and that must therefore be accepted and disguised if necessary with the aid of cosmetics.

Double vision is a rare complication caused by accidental injury to one of the small muscles of the eye controlling its fine movement. The muscle generally heals within a few months, however, thereby restoring synchronous movement and normal binocular vision. Blindness, on the other hand, which has been reported as a consequence of lower eyelid reduction, does not usually have such a happy outcome, although there have also been reports of its successful treatment and reversal. Even though it is excessively rare (estimated to occur once every 500,000 blepharoplasties), it is certainly a complication that a patient should take into account when considering surgery.

Giving Oriental Eyes a Western Look

Partly through the widespread influence of Western television, films and fashion journals, a Western appearance has come to be regarded as desirable in certain Oriental societies and notably among the Japanese, many of whom have adopted Western sports, clothes, hairstyles and various social habits. A few take the rejection of their cultural background further, actually changing their features by surgery of the nose or eyelids in order to enhance their social or professional standing. In areas such as Hawaii, and in Western countries where there is a significant population of Eastern immigrants, Oriental to Occidental surgery has now become relatively commonplace.

The two main differences between the Oriental and Western eyelid lie in the upper lid. That of the Oriental is fuller, lacks a horizontal fold and, where it joins the soft tissue at the inner corner of the eye, ends in an oblique fold of skin called the epicanthus or Mongolian fold, which gives the eye its typical slant. The eyelid as a whole is transformed by modifying just these two characteristics.

The Operation

The preparations, operating conditions, post-operative care and complications of this particular operation are much the same as for general reductive blepharoplasty. A horizontal incision in the upper lid allows the surplus fat lying in front of and beneath the sphincteric muscle of the eyelid to be removed, reducing the overall bulk and leaving redundant eyelid skin which can then be appropriately resected. The next step is to fix the undersurface of the skin to the upper surface of the muscle that opens the eyelid to create the normal Occidental crease and to give a more open eye at rest. The orientation of the Mongolian fold can then be changed by means of a procedure known as a Z-plasty, which is certainly effective but which leaves an unavoidable Z-shaped scar that has to go through all the usual phases of scar maturation (see Fig. 21).

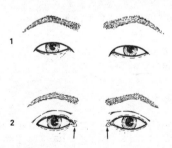

Fig. 21 Making Oriental eyes (1) look more Western involves elevating the upper lids, creating a typical fold and modifying the epicanthus. A small Z-shaped scar is left in the corner of each eye (2).

Eyebrow and Forehead Lift

Horizontal and vertical frown lines can be changed only by a forehead lift and not by the traditional facelift. Although the procedure has been available for many years it has become increasingly popular in recent times as a result of minor innovations that have made it simple, quick, effective and safe, ensuring rapid recovery with no major complications. The operation can be performed under local anaesthesia and leaves a scar that is concealed entirely in the hair-bearing skin of the scalp. In other words a forehead lift has all the attributes one could wish of a cosmetic operation.

The lift is carried out before any upper eyelid reduction as its stretching effect on the eyelid folds can sometimes make blepharoplasty totally unnecessary. The operation is generally most suitable for women, since in men the risk of the post-operative scar, which starts in the hair just above the ears and stretches from ear to ear over the top of the head, becoming exposed as they grow bald in later years is usually unacceptable. In their case an eyebrow lift is the only answer to the problem. The surgical incision is essentially an upward extension of the normal facelift incision (see Fig. 22), so that a forehead lift can easily be added to a facelift without inordinately prolonging the total operating time.

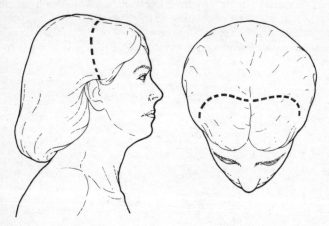

Fig. 22 The browlift incision extends the facelift incision upwards over the top of the head and thus lies conveniently within the hair-bearing area, where the ensuing scar is easy to conceal.

The front of the scalp and the whole of the forehead including the muscle and skin are peeled away, down to the bony ridges underlying the eyebrows. The two small muscles at the top of the nose and between the eyebrows responsible for the vertical frown lines are excised, together with a horizontal strip of the stronger forehead-wrinkling muscle (this does not mean that the patient will no longer be able to wrinkle her forehead but rather that the muscle pull will be diminished, thereby discouraging the return of deep lines). The forehead skin is then pulled tightly upwards so that the excess skin can be measured off and trimmed, after which the skin

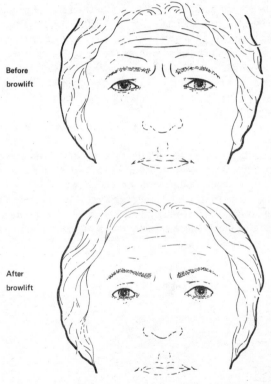

Before
browlift

After
browlift

Fig. 23 The aim of a browlift is to raise the eyebrows into a more pleasing position and to reduce the number and depth of the wrinkles between the eyebrows and on the forehead. A higher brow is usually also obtained.

margins are brought together with stout sutures or staples. Although the skin furrows cannot be completely eliminated by this method, they are satisfactorily flattened out and can be yet further improved by derma-brasion or chemical peel (see Fig. 23). The patient usually returns home the next morning and can wash her hair free of any crusts and debris on the second or third day. The sutures are removed about a week later.

Blood clots (haematomas) under the skin are unlikely to form as the scalp lies tautly over the convex bony vault of the skull, allowing little space for blood to collect and making drains unnecessary. The main problem is numbness at the front of the scalp caused by damage to nerves during the operation. Recovery takes up to twelve months and, like the return of sensation in the face after a facelift, is heralded by a slightly disagreeable tingling. Occasionally the main sensory nerves emerging from small holes in the skull and extending to the eyebrows are also injured, in which case the forehead as well as the scalp loses all feeling for a year. Injury of the hair follicles sufficient to produce a small area of balding is rare, but when it occurs is not permanent, the hair starting to grow again after six months.

A disadvantage rather than a complication is that excision of excess skin causes the frontal hairline to recede by about two or three centimetres – an exchange that most women are happy to make for a smoother forehead. However, if the patient is unhappy at the thought of a higher brow the incision can be made along the hairline itself, whose position will thus remain unchanged after the lift. The price for this, however, is a linear scar and an unnaturally sharp margin to the hairline giving the impression of a wig, disadvantages that generally make surgeons recommend a cut within the hair-bearing area.

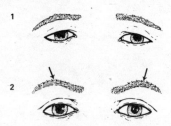

Fig. 24 Drooping eyebrows (1) are corrected by lifting the outer three quarters of each brow via an incision in the upper margin (2). Any bagginess of the eyelids is improved at the same time.

Where patients are concerned only about their drooping eyebrows and have no wish for a full forehead lift, an eyebrow lift alone can be performed. The incision is made just within the upper margin of the eyebrow and a suitable amount of skin excised, so that when the gap is closed the eyebrow is lifted into a more pleasing position (see Fig. 24). To prevent recurrence of the droop, deep permanent sutures are placed beneath the eyebrow, anchoring it to the underlying muscles and deeper tissues in its new site. A fine scar is left which can be covered by brushing the eyebrows upwards and outwards or by using make-up.

[16]

Abdominoplasty and Body Contouring

Abdominoplasty

Pregnancy can permanently mark a woman's figure, leaving a legacy of stretch-marks, slackened breasts and folds of skin overhanging the swollen 'pot' of toneless abdominal muscles referred to by the chauvinistic French male as *la poignée d'amour* (literally 'handful of love'). The same phenomena may equally follow the rigorous self-discipline of months of dieting for overweight, while age and gravity inevitably cause the abdomen slowly to lose its form and flat profile. Abdominoplasty is generally very successful in correcting these effects and has consequently become one of the most frequently performed cosmetic operations, to the great benefit of those women who find that the quality of their lives has become seriously impaired by what they regard as an ugly defect. Many of the procedures used in abdominoplasty as well as in buttock and limb contouring have evolved in North and South America, where to have the body in the smallest bikini means instant success. One need only look at the physiques so flamboyantly paraded on the beaches of Copacabana and Ipanema to understand why the plastic surgeons in Rio de Janeiro are among the busiest cosmetic surgeons in the world.

Like any cosmetic operation, abdominoplasty has its complications and trade-offs which must be fully understood. Marking the skin with a felt-tip pen can give the patient a good idea of the position and extent of the incision, which starts high on the outer side of the thigh, crosses over the top of the leg into the groin and continues up and over the pubic hair-bearing region to join an identical incision from the opposite side, the whole lying within the usual panty or bikini area. An effective abdominoplasty cannot be achieved without extensive scarring, and if a woman is unenthusiastic at the prospect she should not proceed with what is, after all, a major procedure requiring thorough pre-operative examination and investigation.

Abdominoplasty is contra-indicated if the patient has recently undergone upper abdominal surgery, for example for gallstones or stomach ulcers, since the resulting scars jeopardize the blood supply to the skin for at least a year until they have matured. Stretch-marks and recent scars on the *lower* abdomen, however, such as those left after removal of an appendix or ovarian cyst, are included in the area of skin removed during an abdominoplasty and do not constitute such a risk. Surgery is likewise deferred if the patient is unduly overweight, for the surgeon cannot be expected to remove abdominal fat that could easily be lost by dieting. However, if the patient is left with an unsightly abdominal apron after a planned weight loss, the surgeon will be only too happy to complete the process. A good result in an abdominoplasty is achieved through team effort between the surgeon and the patient, who should neither put on excess weight nor embark on any further pregnancies if the initial improvement is to be maintained.

The Operation and After-care

The skin and fat of the abdomen are separated from the underlying muscles via the incision described above and freed up to the lower margin of the rib cage, leaving only the navel intact, detached from the surrounding skin and preserved on a stout stalk in its original position. The thick abdominal sheet thus obtained is then stretched out to its full extent, often reaching halfway down the thighs, and redundant skin and fat excised as necessary. The muscular bulge responsible for the 'pot belly' is flattened by plicating and tightening the abdominal muscles with thick, permanent sutures, after which the skin is securely closed and a small hole cut out over the umbilical stalk so that the navel can be pulled through and sutured into place. Usually the circular defect marking the original site of the navel can be pulled down as far as the pubis, thereby easily fitting into the planned horizontal scar, but if this proves impossible the hole is lengthened into a short vertical cut and sutured to form a midline scar that may unfortunately be less easy to conceal than the main incision (see Fig. 25).

The essential ingredients of abdominoplasty are therefore removal of excess skin and fat, tightening of the muscles (not, however, necessary where the patient is a man or a childless woman undergoing surgery after weight loss), and relocation of the navel.

The patient is sometimes placed in a slightly jack-knifed position on the

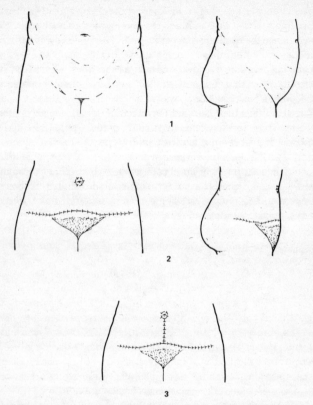

Fig. 25 Abdominoplasty consists of excising redundant skin and fat (1), re-inforcing slack abdominal muscles, and re-siting the navel. A low, long horizontal scar is left (2), sometimes with a vertical extension running upwards to the navel (3), itself surrounded by a small circular scar.

operating table so that the surgeon can achieve an even tighter abdominal repair, and she will find it more comfortable in the following days to maintain this position by sitting up with the knees bent and supported by pillows and by adopting a stoop when walking until the muscles have stretched a little, which they usually do within a week. It is important for the patient to get out of bed as soon as possible, preferably on the next day, in order to prevent one of the most serious complications of any abdominal operation, namely clotting of blood in the deep veins of the legs with its accompanying risk of pulmonary embolism, caused by the clot being swept into the larger vessels of the lungs. Fortunately this has never been a common disaster, and the practice of making the patient get up in the early post-operative stages has made it even rarer. No less than two and frequently four drains are left in the undermined quadrants of the abdomen for at least two days to reduce the chance of a haematoma forming in the abdomen itself. Occasionally the patient is unable to pass urine on the first day and may need to have a catheter passed into the bladder to provide relief, but once she is on her feet its function is restored and the catheter can be withdrawn.

If there is enough help at home from relatives or friends the patient can leave hospital three days later with a tight bandage supporting her abdomen. This is removed together with the sutures after ten to twelve days, and although from now on the patient can straighten up without pain and walk more naturally, she should allow herself at least three weeks' break from work and no less than six weeks before resuming more vigorous activities.

Complications

In 2 per cent of abdominoplasties excess blood collects between the muscles and skin of the abdomen in spite of drains or soon after their removal. This has to be evacuated as an emergency procedure in order to prevent the skin from sloughing. Minor sloughing occurs roughly with the same incidence but is managed without active interference, nature repairing the damage in the course of a few weeks.

The nerves lying at either end of the horizontal incision and serving the outer thighs are sometimes injured during the operation to leave the relevant areas numb or tingling. As the nerves eventually heal, normal feeling returns, but the interval may vary from a few months to as much as one year. If there are no signs of improvement at the end of this time minor surgery via the same incision may be necessary in order to repair the nerves or release them from encasing scar tissue. While damage to these major nerves occurs only rarely, injury of a large number of small sensory nerves is an inevitable part of the undermining process, and leaves a wide belt of numbness or reduced sensation above the scar in the abdominal area. Fortunately this is not a permanent effect, and full recovery is achieved within a year.

The circular scar left around the navel is unattractive and can distort the latter by subsequent contracture. As the scar softens, its appearance generally improves, but in any case revision is a simple matter. Equally simple is readjustment of the navel if it proves obviously off-centre, the only drawback being an additional scar. Perhaps of greater significance to the patient is complete loss of the navel, which occurs (fortunately only rarely) when the blood supply of the umbilicus is cut off during surgery. While the patient might reasonably consider this to be a disaster, it is not however a great problem for the surgeon to create a new navel, which in some instances actually looks better than the old one. So much so that some surgeons in fact prefer to remove the umbilicus as part of the abdominoplasty and make a deep skin dimple instead, which both looks better than the original and entails minimal surface scarring. This aspect of the operation is obviously discussed beforehand with the patient, who may not always be happy to lose such an intimate link with her past.

Body Contouring

It is always bitterly disappointing for the woman who has taken pains to lose a large amount of weight to be left with ugly folds of redundant skin hanging from her thighs, arms and buttocks. Gravity and the ageing process often achieve the same effect, and in the woman who already has heavy thighs and buttocks the additional sagging can be extremely depressing. A source of perhaps even greater frustration is grossly uneven distribution of body fat, which dieting unfortunately cannot help. Whatever the problem, and as with abdominoplasty, the prospective patient must realize that all reasonable effort must be made on her part to lose weight before surgery, since the surgeon cannot be expected to remove fat deposited by over-eating.

Reducing the Buttocks and Thighs

To give the patient a clearer idea of what is involved in surgery of the buttocks and thighs, the surgeon usually marks the position of the incisions on the skin with a felt-tip pen during the preliminary interview. The patient thus has a chance to withdraw from the operation if she finds the extent or location of the cuts unacceptable. Thorough medical assessment is an essential part of the proceedings, as with any major procedure involving general anaesthesia.

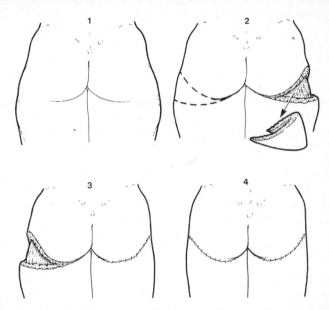

Fig. 26 Heavy buttocks and upper thighs (1) can be reduced by excising large 'melon slices' of fat and skin (2, 3). A long scar is left on each side, stretching from the buttock crease towards the hip-bone (4).

Where reduction of the buttocks and upper thighs is concerned, the surgeon excises an ellipse of skin and fat (the muscles are untouched in this case) from the lower part of the buttocks and the upper thighs, the resulting wound lying along the natural crease between the buttocks and thighs and extending outwards and upwards towards the hip-bones (see Fig. 26). The subsequent scar is easy to conceal as it lies within the panty area.

Excess fat and skin on the inner thighs is also excised as a large ellipse, the incision this time occupying the crease of the groin and sometimes running halfway down the thighs (see Fig. 27).

Drains are used for two days, and although there is some pain during this time the patient is encouraged with the help of suitable pain-killers to take short supervised walks round the room. Stress on the suture lines can be harmful at this stage, and the patient is discouraged from sitting

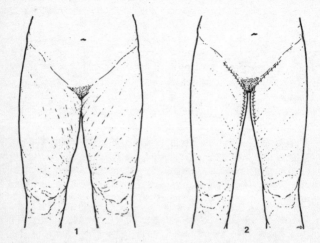

Fig. 27 Excision of redundant fat and skin from the inner thighs (1) leaves scars in the crease of the groin which occasionally extend down the thighs (2).

too long until the sutures have been removed after twelve to fourteen days. As one of the problems following thigh reduction is wound infection secondary to contamination from anal and urinary functions, it is not only permissible but positively beneficial to take a warm salt bath daily from the third day onwards, preferably lying rather than sitting throughout. If infection does occur, it is treated with antibiotics and local dressings. The only other early complication is a haematoma, which as always is removed as quickly as possible. The patient can return to work after three weeks and resume all her usual activities after six.

The commonest long-term problem is slight separation of the layer of fat immediately beneath the scar, leading to the formation of a shallow dent, easily visible under tight clothes. Unfortunately this is difficult to avoid or treat effectively, even if an overlapping layer of fat is incorporated.

Surgery to remove fat from the knees or from heavy calves is not recommended, since the results are disappointing and the scars likely to attract more attention than the original condition.

Arm Reduction

The matronly, flabby upper arm can be an embarrassment in young women who have recently lost weight, as well as in the middle-aged and elderly. Women with this type of disfigurement, commonly known as a 'bat-wing deformity', will probably avoid stretching movements in public that display the swaying, hanging curtains of skin folds and fat, try to keep their arms by their sides, and select clothes with sleeves extending below the elbow.

Treatment for flabbiness in the upper arms is both safe and easy, has no immediate untoward complications and requires a stay of only one night in hospital, but unfortunately the resulting scar is so long, extending from the armpit to just above the elbow (see Fig. 28), that a woman who was originally self-conscious about her fleshy arms may now be self-conscious about her scars. The patient must judge for herself if the exchange is worthwhile.

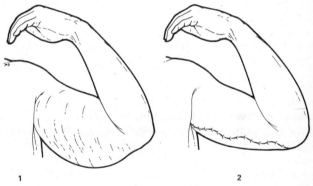

1   2

Fig. 28 Excess skin and fat in the region of the upper arms (1) is cut out to leave a sinuous scar running from the armpit to the elbow (2).

Limb and Buttock Augmentation

In the past, women who objected to their skinny calves could not be helped, but a technique has now been developed whereby custom-designed silicone implants can be used to augment the calves via a hori-zontal incision behind the knee leading to a pocket in the calf. The immediate results look impressive, but unfortunately walking, running and fibrous encapsulation (see pp. 142–4) tend to displace the prostheses, so that the majority in fact have to be removed if they have not already eroded through the skin. This type of surgery has not won any acclaim in Britain, where the more conservative cosmetic surgeons regard it as unwarranted and unjustifiable. Women genuinely disturbed by the spindly appearance of their legs would be better advised to follow the example of fifteenth-century courtiers and wear suitable padding under their stockings.

A group of South American surgeons has also described how to augment the buttocks by inserting a breast prosthesis into each cheek through a cut made in the buttock crease. Although this treatment is looked at askance by certain north European surgeons, it is simple, safe and apparently satisfies the customer. No doubt the pressure of sitting makes for permanently soft and mobile prostheses, thereby preventing encapsulation – a distinct advantage, and one not encountered in other forms of prosthetic augmentation.

Fat Suction

A major disadvantage of abdominal, thigh and buttock reduction is obviously the extensive scarring entailed. In an effort to keep this to a minimum, other means of body contouring have been devised. One which enjoyed a brief vogue consisted of removing fat via a small incision with the help of an instrument rather like a long-handled ladle with a sharp margin to its bowl. Using this the surgeon scooped fat out of the thighs or buttocks, sometimes thinning it beforehand with a sterilized, long-spindled whisk which churned the thick lumps into a mixture that could be more readily spooned. Unfortunately, not just fat but other structures such as arteries, veins and nerves were also removed, and the technique was eventually abandoned.

In the last few years a comparable system has been introduced whereby fat is aspirated under high negative pressure through long metal cannulae or tubes inserted into the relevant anatomical area. The proponents of this technique claim that fat and nothing but fat is removed. They also propose, quite reasonably, that there are two different types of fat. The first fluctuates in volume according to dietary habits; while it can be reduced simply by dieting, it re-forms on over-eating. The other, which can be regarded as a hereditary trait, tends to remain unchanged regardless of food intake and is deposited mainly below the waist, especially around the buttocks, hips and upper thighs. Once removed, this type of fat is unlikely to re-form, and is therefore best suited to aspiration.

Fat suction is neither suitable for all patients nor without its problems. Following experience with several hundred patients, the leading practitioners in France suggest that the best candidates are women with excess fat around the hips but no skin redundancy and who are under thirty-five years of age, since as a result of the reduced skin tone in women over forty the skin does not lie well over the underlying tissues once the fat has been aspirated and hangs in small festoons which require surgical excision, a procedure leaving the very same long scars that the patient wished to avoid in the first place. Indeed, a middle-aged woman with what is described as a 'riding-breeches deformity' (i.e., heavy thighs) may well find herself with a 'golfing plus-fours deformity' after the fat has been sucked out. It therefore follows that both older women and those with excess skin and fat or the unacceptable consequences of pregnancy or weight loss are not suitable for fat suction and can be treated only by the traditional methods already described.

The Operation and Complications
The areas to be aspirated are marked out beforehand with the patient standing up. Half an hour before the procedure a dilute salt solution is injected under the skin, disrupting the membranes around the fat cells and converting the fat into a liquefied form that can be more easily aspirated. The procedure is carried out under general anaesthesia by means of a long metal cannula connected to a vacuum pump and inserted into the fat pad via a one-centimetre incision made in a natural skin crease and at some distance from the area to be de-fatted. The vacuum pump is switched on and the fat sucked out as a yellow sludge into a calibrated glass container allowing the surgeon to measure its volume. Not more than two kilograms can be safely removed at one time and if further suction is required it must be left to another session. Drains are then inserted into the emptied fat pocket, where they are left for about two days. After this time the patient can be sent home, the treated areas firmly bandaged for a fortnight in order to reduce the inevitable bruising and swelling, which can persist for up to six or eight weeks if not relieved by massage and physiotherapy. The patient is advised to rest at home for two weeks and return to a normal lifestyle only after six.

The main complaint of women undergoing fat suction is firstly that it is painful and makes walking difficult for about a month, and secondly that a slightly shelving defect is left at the periphery of the aspirated zone where it meets the full thickness of normal body fat. An occasional specific complication appears to be infection of the aspiration site together with partial sloughing of the skin following over-vigorous suction.

Although high-vacuum fat suction has so far been described by its advocates only in an anecdotal fashion and has not met with much enthusiasm within the surgical establishment, the technique is slowly gaining ground and already there are reports from southern Europe and South America of the use of fat suction in ankle, calf, arm, breast and abdominal reduction and in the removal of facial fat. However, in the more conservative arena of northern Europe, and even in North America, surgeons, many of whom perhaps find it difficult to picture themselves, after their many years of training in highly complex reconstructive surgery, holding a metal pipe inserted into a podgy hip while a sophisticated vacuum cleaner sucks fat into a glass jar, will doubtless remain cynical until the method has been subjected to the usual rigorous and objective clinical analysis.

[17]

Changing the Shape of Breasts

In surgical breast augmentation, reduction and reconstruction, the goal is to help women whose lives are genuinely disturbed by a real or imagined defect in their breasts or who simply dislike them on cosmetic grounds and wish to change them. A brief discussion of the structure and function of the breasts may help the patient firstly to understand what changes are possible and secondly how these are achieved.

Essentially the breast is a skin appendage lying on a broad muscular base and composed of multiple milk-secreting glands from which ducts emerge on to the surface via the nipple (see Fig. 29). The firmness of the breast is ensured by the fibrous tissue encasing the gland tubes, while the normal cone shape is due to the convergence of milk-carrying ducts on the nipple. The latter is surrounded by an area of pigmented skin covered with small nodules (called Montgomery tubercles after the anatomist who

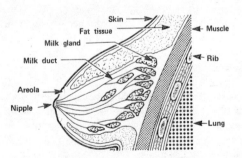

Fig. 29 The breast is basically a collection of milk glands and ducts contained within an envelope of fat and skin and surmounted by a nipple/areola complex. The foundation is a thick layer of muscle overlying the ribs.

first described them) known as the areola, which together with the nipple is provided with small muscles that erect the nipple when the nerves are stimulated by an outside source. The whole glandular system is contained within an envelope of skin similar to that overlying the abdomen and chest.

At its simplest, therefore, the breast is a bag of skin containing a mass of soft tissue and thus a structure relatively easy to modify. The possibilities for change are various: if the contents are too small they can be increased; if the sac is too slack but the contents are of normal volume the skin can be tightened; if the entire structure is too large it can be reduced; if the breasts are unequal they can be matched; and if one has been lost due to mastectomy for cancer it can be restored, although never in its original form. Even the nipple, if inverted or if it does not project as desired, can be corrected. Cosmetic surgery of the breast is seldom performed before the age of eighteen unless the breasts are grotesquely enormous. Where older women are concerned, the surgeon's decision as to the feasibility of an operation is made on the basis of the patient's health, physical make-up and motivation. Age itself is not a barrier.

Breast Augmentation

The size of the breasts depends on genetic and hormonal factors alike: a woman may have unusually small breasts as part of her genetic inheritance or develop small or even smaller breasts as a result of hormonal influence on the breast tissue after the menopause or the birth of a child. Whatever the case, augmentation of the breasts is one of the two most common operations in women, and an estimated 30,000 female patients undergo breast augmentation each year in the USA, the leading cosmetic-surgical consumer country in the world. This figure undoubtedly owes much to the introduction of the silicone prosthesis.

Before the 1960s the materials used in augmentation were the patient's own tissues, taken either from the abdomen or from the buttocks as a large graft of fat and skin. The operation was time-consuming, tedious, fraught with complications, and left ugly scars and defects in the donor area, so that plastic surgeons were delighted, in the early 1960s, to abandon the method and turn instead to silicone.

Chemically and physically the silicones are fascinating. They vary in consistency from an oily liquid to a solid block; they are heat-stable, deteriorate very slowly and are therefore suitable for prolonged implantation in human tissue; they are non-toxic and cannot be linked in any way with cancer. No woman thinking of breast augmentation thus need fear breast cancer as a side-effect of the operation. Despite being biologically inert, however, silicone implants are not without their problems, as will later become apparent.

Breast prostheses, which make use of high-grade medical silicone, generally consist of a relatively firm outer shell and a soft, jelly-like core, and at body temperature have a consistency and mobility identical to that of breast tissue. The typical prosthesis has a circular base and a fairly low profile, and resembles nothing more than a stranded jellyfish. Other shapes have been introduced in the hope of changing the outline of the breast as well as increasing its volume, but although spherical, pear-shaped, teardrop-shaped and cone-shaped implants have all had their vogue, none have succeeded in achieving this aim. Alternatively the prosthesis may consist of an inflatable silicone bag, which in its collapsed state has the advantage that it can be inserted through a very small hole before being inflated through a valvular tube with sterile water. Although the occasional bag does later leak, thereby collapsing the breast, this is a rare complication and the inflatable prosthesis is still favoured by many plastic surgeons. .

Silicone injected in its soft, oily state must never be used to increase the volume of the breast. The complications in terms of pain, infection, ulceration, distortion and displacement are disastrous, but unfortunately continue to be seen as a result of the work of unscrupulous, untrained, non-medical practitioners.

How does the surgeon determine the right size of prosthesis for a given woman? Measurement and objective assessment are not particularly useful in this case, and the decision relies more on subjective criteria such as the surgeon's experience, the patient's preferences and the dictates of fashion. The range of prostheses currently on the market varies in increments of 20 cc from 100 to 460 cc, but since most women requesting augmentation are slim and therefore not built for very large breasts, the surgeon generally advises a prosthesis of 120 to 180 cc (200 to 280 cc in the USA, where fashion favours larger breasts). A woman who already has a large bust but even so desires augmentation, will need a correspondingly large prosthesis to provide the necessary increase in bulk, and one of up to 360 cc may be used in this case. Should the patient want a more accurate assessment, a fairly good method is to insert various prostheses between her breast and the cup of a bra she wishes to fill until the one most suitable for the purpose is found. This can then be used in the operation.

It should perhaps be mentioned at this point that while there is no evidence whatsoever of a link between breast augmentation and breast cancer, the latter is unfortunately so common in women (one in seventeen can expect to develop breast cancer in their lifetime) that it is normal practice to check not just the patient's health overall before surgery but also to make a careful examination of the breasts for lumps or other signs of cancer. If a lump is found, further investigations of the type described in Chapter 8 will be carried out to ascertain its nature. As far as screening after breast augmentation is concerned, patients can be reassured that the implant will be placed deep in the breast and that subsequent detection of lumps will therefore not be hampered.

In the UK, the operation is generally carried out under general anaesthesia and involves a stay of at least twenty-four hours in hospital.

The Operation and After-care

The operation basically consists of creating a pocket beneath the breast that will accommodate the prosthesis. Depending on the surgeon's preference, this will be made either between the front of the chest muscle and the undersurface of the breast or between the ribs and the undersurface of the muscle (see Fig. 30), neither method interfering with the milk-

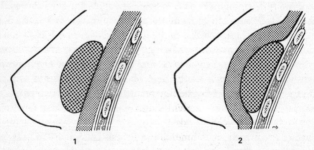

Fig. 30 Breast augmentation is achieved by placing a suitably sized silicone prosthesis either between the muscle and the breast tissue (1) or between the muscle and the ribs (2).

secreting glands or with the duct system and therefore with breastfeeding. The incision is commonly made in the lower half of the breast just above the crease where the breast joins the chest or, less frequently, within the rim of the areola itself or behind the fold forming the front wall of the armpit (see Fig. 31).

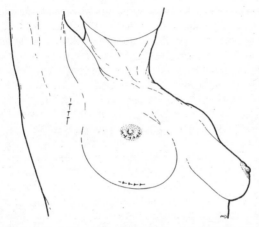

Fig. 31 The prosthesis is usually inserted via an incision just above the crease in the lower part of the breast. Less frequently the cut is made in the armpit or within the areola.

Separation of the tissues inevitably causes a small amount of bleeding, and while a few surgeons leave this to be absorbed through the walls of the pocket, most prefer to draw off the blood by means of a small drain, inserted in the breast and removed the following day. Bandages are worn for a period of seven to ten days to support the breasts, and during this time the patient is advised not to stretch her arms or lift heavy objects. The sutures are removed at the end of this time, together with the bandages. It is usual for the patient to return to work after two weeks and to resume normal physical activities after four; she can also start to go braless from this point onwards if she likes. Some surgeons advocate massage of the breasts, recommending that patients push the prosthesis up towards the collar-bone and inwards towards the breast-bone for ten minutes twice daily for up to six weeks in an effort to prevent the pocket from contracting and hardening (see 'Complications', overleaf).

Complications

Very rarely, leaking blood fills the pocket containing the prosthesis and clots to produce painful ballooning of the breasts. Although this complication is very infrequent and in fact occurs only in about 1 per cent of all patients, it justifies a speedy return to the operating theatre for evacuation of the clot, sealing of any bleeding points and re-insertion of the prosthesis.

Infection, which is equally rare, can be effectively treated only by removing the prosthesis, prescribing antibiotics and waiting for the tissue reaction to settle. The interval between removal and safe replacement of the prosthesis seldom amounts to less than three months, and although it may be difficult for the disappointed patient to accept the necessity of the corrective treatment, unless the prosthesis is immediately removed it may actually fall out through the incision, since if this is left to become infected it will eventually break down and gape open.

In one out of ten women, certain sensory nerves leading from the nipple are damaged during the operation, resulting in reduced sensation or, occasionally, in painful hypersensitivity. There is unfortunately little that can be done to restore normal sensation, and all the patient can do is avoid physical contact with the nipple as far as possible in the latter case and wait up to six months for the nerves to recover.

Some degree of asymmetry in breast size and shape is natural and inevitable, but if the prostheses are incorrectly balanced the variation may become unacceptable. Obviously a surgeon takes all the necessary precautions to avoid the problem, but even so prostheses that are carefully positioned in their pockets when the patient is lying supine on the operating table sometimes appear lopsided when she eventually stands up. Massage and manipulation will not correct the asymmetry, and the only solution is to perform corrective surgery and reposition the prostheses.

By far the most frequent and worst-understood complication is capsular contracture or fibrous encapsulation, which occurs in 10 to 40 per cent of patients according to various estimates. The process involves a gradual accumulation of fibrous tissue around the prosthesis until a stage is reached where the latter not only becomes firm and loses its natural mobility but may become as hard as a cricket ball. The force exerted by the contracting and encircling scar simultaneously distorts the prosthesis, causing the breast to develop into an ugly, tender sphere (see Fig. 32).

Every plastic surgeon is acutely aware of the problem, and although

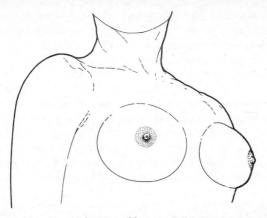

Fig. 32 The commonest complication of breast augmentation is excessive scar encapsulation of the prostheses, distorting the breasts into hard, tender spheres.

hardly a plastic-surgical journal is published without yet another method for reducing the chances of capsular contracture being described, there is as yet no perfect solution. Nor, unfortunately, are there any means of telling which patients are likely to develop hard breasts after augmentation. In the meantime, if a woman wishes to have her breasts enlarged, she has no choice but to accept both the risk of hardening and the fairly primitive methods used to treat it.

One of these, described as 'breast popping', was found by chance when a patient suffering from capsular contracture after augmentation was inadvertently punched on the hardened breast, which softened immediately and painfully with a cracking noise. The woman consulted her surgeon, who in exploring the breast discovered that the encircling scar had split open and that the prosthesis was now lying in its original shape and position. The treatment has since been advocated of splitting the capsule by powerfully squeezing the whole sphere between two fists until it cracks and the breast softens, the patient being sedated or anaesthetized throughout. Perhaps surprisingly, it is always the capsule that breaks, never the prosthesis itself. If the surgeon is unable to obtain sufficient grasp to break the capsule, the breast must be opened and the latter split directly, the pocket being enlarged at the same time. Whatever the method, the breast is tender for a few days and occasionally a lump may be noticed where part of the prosthesis has herniated through a narrow split to bulge out into the breast tissue. If this happens the surgical wound is reopened and the split completed by direct incision of the capsule. Unfortunately the correction is not permanent: it is not unusual for recontracture to occur within six months, although it is usually less pronounced than in the first instance.

A woman thinking of undergoing what she has up till now believed to be a simple procedure to increase the size of her bust may be a little discouraged by the possible prospect of acquiring certainly larger but harder and misshapen breasts with a detectable scar, but on the positive side only 10 to 40 per cent of women requesting breast augmentation experience capsular contracture: the rest come safely through the operation with larger, better-shaped and naturally soft and mobile breasts.

Breast Reduction

Apart from the embarrassment that over-large, pendulous breasts cause many women, their great bulk makes for discomfort, pain and various other physical problems. For example, even if a woman can find a comfortable bra the load suspended from the straps digs tender and sometimes permanent grooves in her shoulders; the postural compensation necessary to offset the weight of the breasts can, in the long term, lead to a stoop with arthritic changes in the vertebral column of the neck; and the underside of the breasts often becomes infected due to moisture collecting between the breasts and the chest and upper abdomen, ending in a situation where fungal infection converts the moistened skin to a sore, red, malodorous surface comparable to that seen in athlete's foot. Surgery to make the breasts smaller is thus not merely a cosmetic procedure but also a very useful treatment which, in the case of certain women with enormous breasts, actually prevents or resolves pain and associated diseases.

The Operation and After-care

Complete physical examination and medical investigation before surgery are essential as the operation is a major one, lasting up to three hours and requiring general anaesthesia. The procedure is complex, but basically consists of dismantling the breast, shifting the nipple and areola to a higher position, excising the excess breast tissue and skin and re-assembling what remains into a smaller, more compact shape (see Fig. 33).

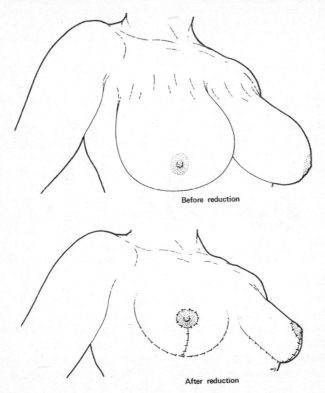

Before reduction

After reduction

Fig. 33 Breast reduction essentially consists of dismantling the breasts, removing excess tissue, elevating the nipple and areola and reassembling the remaining tissues. With the exception of the cut around the areola, all the incisions are made in the lower half of the breasts.

Careful planning of the operation is as important as technique, and for this reason the surgeon starts by marking out a pattern of measured lines, points and angles on the surface of the breast as an aid to achieving a more accurate and symmetrical result. Although various methods exist, two basic techniques are used, each characterized by different drawbacks and complications.

In the first the nipple and areola are carried up on a flap of breast tissue

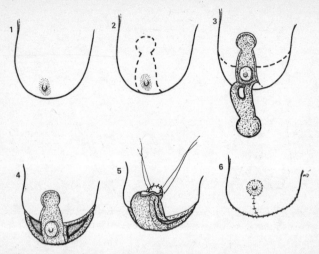

Fig. 34 The most common method of breast reduction is excision of redundant tissue followed by elevation of the nipple/areola complex on a flap of tissue carrying its own blood and nerve supply.

containing a rich blood supply and nerve plexus (or network of nerves) but are separated from the milk-carrying ducts in the process (see Fig. 34).

In the second the nipple and areola are removed completely from the duct system, its blood supply and the nerve plexus and repositioned as a free graft higher up on a prepared bed of breast tissue (see Fig. 35).

The first technique is used for moderately large breasts, the second for enormous breasts or where the blood flow within a nipple-carrying flap is likely to be unpredictable. Whichever method is used to relocate the nipple the final position of the suture lines is the same, resulting in a fine circumferential scar around the re-sited areola, a vertical scar from its lower pole to the crease of the breast, and a curved horizontal scar hidden within the full length of the crease between the breast and the chest.

To prevent too much blood from accumulating within the breasts after surgery, narrow drainage tubes are usually left inside for one or two days to drain off the excess into two small bottles. Patients can return home on the second or third day wearing firm supporting bandages, removed together with all the sutures after ten to twelve days, and resume their

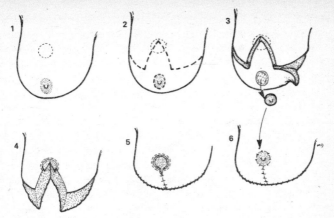

Fig. 35 If the breasts are very large and pendulous, the nipple and areola are removed as a graft and relocated after the excess tissue has been removed.

daily routine after about a fortnight, although they should avoid sports and any comparable activities for at least six weeks.

Complications

Since drains are unable to cope with heavy bleeding, blood clots, which painfully distend the breasts, are a possibility. As in breast augmentation, facelift or any other cosmetic procedure, large haematomas seriously threaten the success of the operation and are therefore evacuated in the operating theatre as a matter of urgency. This complication occurs in about 2 per cent of all breast reductions.

Partial sloughing of the areola and nipple is similarly infrequent and results in the formation of a scab, which falls off once new tissue has grown beneath it. The resulting surface is always much paler, giving the areola a permanent piebald appearance. Very rarely the blood supply within the nipple/areola-bearing flap is inadequate and the areola sloughs completely, necessitating reconstruction of the whole complex according to the technique described on p. 158. Women with excessively large breasts whose nipple and areola are relocated as a graft inevitably experience some degree of scabbing, but this is preferable to the complete loss possible with the alternative method.

Minor sloughing of the breast skin itself is not uncommon, particularly in the area of maximum tension where the vertical incision meets the curved, horizontal incision. Once again nature is the best physician, for new skin grows to replace the old within about six weeks, leaving only a pale and not particularly noticeable triangle on the underside of the breast. However, in the much rarer event of a major skin slough, which occurs in less than 1 per cent of patients, the surgeon may be compelled to cut out the dead skin and resurface the area with a skin graft.

10 per cent of patients experience a curious complication called fat necrosis, which is related to disturbance of the blood supply within the breast during its rearrangement and consists of small or large areas of fat growing tender, hard and knobbly in the first few days after surgery as a result of being poorly perfused with blood. The damage generally heals by itself, but the process of replacement is very slow and may take up to six months to reach completion. In the meantime the patient may be a little disturbed to feel hard lumps within her breast, believing them to be a sign of cancer. She can be reassured both that her fears are unfounded and that the tissue removed in the course of breast reduction is always checked by a pathologist to make sure it contains no suspicious foci.

The considerable scarring inevitably resulting from the operation may be regarded by some as a complication but can equally well be seen as a reasonable exchange for unmanageable breasts. Similarly with the reduction or loss of normal and erotic nipple sensation inherent in many techniques. Although this loss is not always acceptable among women with only moderately large breasts, it should be realized that while a surgeon tries to preserve the nerve plexus supplying the nipple/areola complex there can be no guarantee that normal sensation will be preserved – indeed it is usually diminished. The milk-carrying duct system is unfortunately always divided, so that patients can never breastfeed, although there have been isolated reports of the ducts later linking with the nipple even when this has been repositioned as a graft. Flattening or inversion of the nipple occasionally follows reduction but can be corrected relatively easily (see p. 151).

Post-operative asymmetry of the breasts or of the nipple/areola complex considered as falling outside the normal range can later be corrected by relatively minor surgery with the patient as a day or overnight case.

Drooping Breasts

Although breasts engorge and distend during pregnancy, they return to their original volume as soon as breastfeeding comes to an end. Unfortunately the skin encasing them seldom regains its initial tautness. In most women the slackness is of little note, but in some the skin envelope is so baggy and covered with so many stretch-marks that it can constitute a source of considerable embarrassment. There is no explanation for the very variable response of women's skin to pregnancy and no obvious reason why some are adversely affected in this respect and others not at all. What is certain, however, is that the slackness can occasionally be compounded by the effects of gravity and ageing, as the collagen and elastic fibres surrounding the glands of the breast and within the skin itself lose their ability to support the breasts, to the extent where the latter become little more than two flaps of skin hanging loosely from the chest wall. Exactly the same phenomenon can sometimes be seen among women who have lost a lot of weight through dieting.

Treatment consists of excising the redundant skin and tightening the envelope to restore the normal cone shape, but leaving the volume of the breast unchanged. Unfortunately there is no way of treating stretch-marks, although a proportion will be lost along with the excised skin.

Surgery and its Complications

Although the operation is designed along the same lines as breast reduction, with the same pre-operative planning and skin marking, it is not as major an undertaking, since no breast tissue is removed. The patient does not usually remain in hospital longer than one night and drains are seldom required. All the complications, caveats and precautions applicable to breast reduction, apply here, but to a lesser degree. As the nipple is seldom detached from the underlying structures, sensitivity is rarely impaired and the patient may subsequently breastfeed, although it is unlikely she will go through another pregnancy having undergone surgery precisely to mitigate the effects of the first. The scars are similarly sited but do not extend as far along the undersurface of the breast.

While a woman undergoing complete breast reduction will often be delighted to see her new breasts for the first time, a patient who has undergone simple tightening of the skin may not be too thrilled. The reason for this is that the surgeon often over-corrects the slackness, giving a flattened rather than a convex contour to the breasts from the nipples downwards. Over the next three to four weeks, however, the skin stretches sufficiently to restore the natural curve, enhancing yet further the initial improvement.

After a reduction, the breasts, even if they tend gradually to lose their shape, remain unaltered as to size. If the breasts have only been tightened, however, gravity and age slowly overcome the correction. The operation can of course be repeated, but there comes a point at which the patient must give in to inevitability and accept that gravity has won.

Small Drooping Breasts

One might imagine that an undersized breast within an over-large envelope of skin could simply be corrected by inserting a breast prosthesis under the excess skin. Unfortunately, many efforts to do just that create a misshapen breast from which the skin continues to hang in folds, and both breast augmentation and tightening of the skin are therefore necessary to achieve a good shape and size. Since it is not easy to carry out both operations at the same time, many surgeons now perform the correction in two stages separated by six months, the first to remove redundant skin and the second to augment the breast (the two operations have already been described under separate headings). In fact it is surprising how many women find themselves quite happy with the size of their breasts once the shape has been improved and decide not to go ahead with the second stage.

Unequal Breasts

It has already been mentioned that a minor degree of asymmetry is natural, but nature can be unfair and go to extremes. Thus while one woman with unequal breasts may require only a little padding in one cup of her bra, another with virtually no breast, nipple or areola on one side of her body – fortunately a rare occurrence – may need an external prosthesis of the kind used by patients after mastectomy for cancer. In a case of mild asymmetry the patient is left to decide for herself whether to have the larger breast reduced or the smaller breast augmented, but the surgeon, knowing that augmentation is fraught with the risk of fibrous encapsulation and that reducing the larger breast in any case gives a better long-term result, even if the scarring is more extensive, may well try to influence the decision in the former direction. Moderate to severe degrees of asymmetry can be corrected only by internal prosthetic augmentation, while total lack of breast development on one side requires surgical reconstruction similar to that after mastectomy. Rather as in reconstruction, correction of unequal breast volume is reasonably simple, but construction of an entire second breast comparable in shape to the first is not so easy, and a woman may have to come to terms with having equal-sized breasts one of which is a little slacker than the other.

It should be pointed out that an infrequent cause of breast asymmetry is the presence of a tumour in the larger breast, so the patient should be prepared for the necessary investigations and treatment.

Extra Breasts

In rare cases supernumerary breasts may develop, usually in the armpit but occasionally along a line from the normal breasts to the groin and even on the buttocks. Whether they take the form of a diffuse swelling or of a fully grown breast and nipple which produces milk during pregnancy (one classic textbook of surgery contains an illustration showing a baby being suckled from a breast in the groin), they are simple to remove, as is the more common rudimentary extra nipple sometimes seen (both in women and men) on the upper abdomen just below the breast and frequently mistaken for a brown mole.

Inverted Nipples

A potentially embarrassing defect is a flat or inverted nipple on one or both breasts, caused by abnormal shortness of the tethering, underlying milk ducts. Treatment, which is carried out under general or local anaesthesia with the patient as a day case, consists of cutting through the areola or nipple, thus obtaining access to the shortened ducts, parting these so as to free the nipple, and helping the latter to project with the help of a few deep, everting sutures. While the operation is quick, easy, effective and relatively trouble-free, it does unfortunately rule out any possibility of breastfeeding and causes some loss of nipple sensation.

Male Breasts

Not only do all men have nipples and areolas: they also have breast tissue. Although this is not normally obvious as a swelling it may, under hormonal influence, enlarge to an embarrassing size. In fact one in three of all boys around the age of puberty have some degree of breast enlargement (called gynaecomastia, meaning literally 'breast of a woman'), which can occasionally be so pronounced that they will adopt a typical posture, wear loose shirts in order to disguise the swelling and avoid any activity where their chests will be exposed in public. In most cases, fortunately, their breasts will have returned to normal by the end of eighteen months. A small number of young men, however, are left with persistent gynaecomastia; these can, if they wish, undergo surgical treatment.

In older men, breast enlargement is often associated with a disease involving the liver or the hormone-producing glands, or occurs as a side-effect of certain drugs. Treatment here is therefore directed at the underlying cause rather than at the breast tissue itself. Breast cancer can also be a problem, although its incidence is low: only one man for every 200 women develops the disease. The treatment is much the same as in female patients except that the prognosis is worse.

Surgery and Complications

Treatment for gynaecomastia consists of surgical excision of the redundant breast tissue via a cut made within the areola (see Fig. 36). The operation is performed under general anaesthesia and usually involves a stay of at least two days in hospital to allow for adequate drainage of the breast pocket (the commonest early complication is a large haematoma). If there is so much breast tissue that it cannot easily be removed through such a small incision the surgeon is obliged to make a larger cut in the

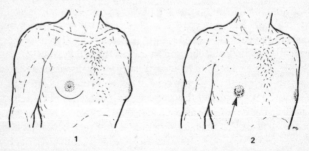

Fig. 36 Excess male breast tissue (1) is removed via a curved incision along the lower rim of the areola. The subsequent scar cannot easily be detected (2).

breast skin itself, which means a more obvious scar. The stitches are taken out after ten days.

It is not easy to remove the breast tissue without also removing some of the underlying fat, and although the surgeon bevels the cut, a shallow, concave defect often remains after the operation. (Fortunately this gradually builds up with fat over the following years and eventually disappears.) Similarly, the nipple, deprived of its support, can become flattened or depressed or even adhere to the underlying muscle. However, judging from the enthusiastic response of patients to the operation, these are minor drawbacks.

Reconstruction of the Breast after Mastectomy

Breast cancer is unfortunately so common that one woman in seventeen can expect to develop the disease during her lifetime. Although radiotherapy and chemotherapy (treatment with drugs) can sometimes, depending on the patient's age and the type of tumour, replace mastectomy as a treatment, the majority of women with breast cancer have part or all of their breast removed, the amount excised varying according to the training and instincts of the surgeon concerned and the characteristics and spread of the tumour. Sadly, despite all the energy, capital and expertise thrown into research on breast cancer, there is still no ideal or universally accepted line of treatment. One surgeon will treat a tumour by simply excising a wedge of breast tissue, preserving the nipple and areola, while another will remove not just the whole breast but also the underlying base of muscles together with the glands in the armpit, and prescribe radiotherapy and chemotherapy into the bargain. As things are at present, neither technique can really be faulted, each having its own currency. What can be criticized, however, is the failure of certain general surgeons to sympathize with the plight of patients having good prospects of survival after the operation and to inform them that reconstruction is possible, let alone refer them to a plastic surgeon to discuss the procedure. The fact that more than 95 per cent of general surgeons are male may have something to do with this lack of understanding, but a reluctance to suggest cosmetic surgery after mastectomy for cancer is often based on the belief – unsubstantiated, let it be said – that reconstruction changes the course of the disease or hinders the detection and subsequent treatment of the tumour if it spreads or recurs. Fortunately attitudes are changing, and the majority of general surgeons readily engage the help of a plastic surgeon. A few even carry out the reconstruction themselves, whether immediately after the mastectomy or after a suitable interval. Gone are the days when the surgeon gave the patient a pat on the back and a prescription for an external prosthesis, and dismissed her with the remark: 'You're lucky to be alive, my dear.'

Thus if a woman with a favourable prognosis who wishes to be considered for reconstruction is faced with an unsympathetic surgeon she has every right to seek another opinion. Nonetheless it must be stressed that the priority in breast cancer is proper and unreserved treatment of the disease itself, and no responsible surgeon will tailor his initial care to cosmetic requirements. It should also be said that if the patient does undergo breast reconstruction, it is important for her to remain under the charge of the original general surgeon or radiotherapist so that he can monitor her progress.

Having experienced one major operation for the treatment of breast cancer not every woman wants to go through another for reconstruction, and the majority in fact accept the residual deformity and external prosthesis worn under the clothing to disguise the defect. A few patients, however, never come to terms with the loss of their breast and remain emotionally and psychologically disturbed. A study by a group of psychiatrists and psychologists found that 40 per cent of women undergoing mastectomy were left with serious anxiety, depression or sexual problems, and that although some were helped by counselling and drugs a few continued to exhibit severe and persistent symptoms; these seemed to be paying an undesirably high price for their better prospects of survival. It was suggested that patients with sexual difficulties could most benefit from reconstructive surgery; and there is in fact no doubt that reconstruction of the breast after mastectomy is invaluable for those women whose quality of life is seriously at risk. However, it is not necessary for women to suffer in order to earn a reconstruction, and the majority seeking this form of surgery have not experienced psychological problems after the mastectomy but are simply fed up with the external prosthesis and the limited choice of clothes.

Surgery and Complications

No one can restore a breast. The surgeon can only construct a more or less convincing mound which matches as closely as possible the characteristics of the opposite breast in terms of siting, shape, colour and skin texture and in the size, projection, colour and position of the nipple/areola complex.

What is the ideal time to reconstruct? As in the treatment of breast cancer itself there are no clear guidelines. Some surgeons believe that breast shape should be restored immediately after mastectomy and as part of the same operation so that the patient can leave hospital fully equipped. Others like to examine the excised tissue and so determine the precise type and extent of the tumour before considering reconstruction and possibly radiotherapy as well. But as a very general rule reconstruction is feasible within six months of mastectomy if no radiotherapy has been used. If it has, reconstruction is delayed for at least a year because radiation has a significantly harmful effect where healing of a wound is concerned.

Reconstruction is basically a matter of surgical arithmetic in which any structures that have been removed are replaced in kind: the more radical the mastectomy the more complex the surgical equation to equalize the result. Thus if a woman has lost the breast but has enough underlying skin and muscle left, an internal prosthesis is all that will be required; the operation will be comparable to a breast augmentation, with similar short- and long-term complications. If, on the other hand, the woman has had an extensive mastectomy in which all the tissues, including the chest muscles, have been removed to leave a tight drum of skin over the chest wall, new skin, muscle and bulk in the form of a prosthesis will all need to be provided.

Where skin and muscle are required, these are commonly taken from the patient's back as a flap, dependent for its survival on a narrow pedicle of muscle, artery and vein connecting it to the back wall of the armpit, and rotated on the axis of the pedicle so as to cover the relevant breast area. Additional bulk is afforded by a silicone prosthesis, which is insulated by the muscles brought over from the back. The old skin, supplemented by the new, provides the envelope for the breast (see Fig. 37).

Alternatively, the bulk (in the form of fat), muscle and skin can be obtained from the lower abdomen, using the same flap technique but no prosthesis (see Fig. 38). Although this method has two advantages, firstly that all the problems encountered with the silicone prosthesis, and particularly that of fibrous encapsulation, are avoided, and secondly that a patient with a sagging abdomen has the added bonus of an abdomino-plasty, unfortunately complications are more frequent with an abdominal flap than with a back flap.

Since reconstruction of the breast using large flaps is a major surgical

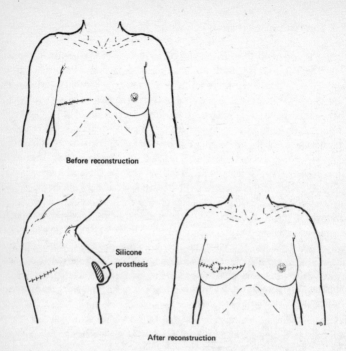

Before reconstruction

Silicone prosthesis

After reconstruction

Fig. 37 If, after mastectomy, the breast mound cannot be reconstructed by prosthetic augmentation alone, new tissue in the form of skin and muscle can be transferred from the back to the breast region as a flap. A silicone prosthesis can then be added to make the reconstruction complete.

undertaking lasting not less than two hours and requiring up to seven days' hospitalization, it is essential for the patient to know all the risks and drawbacks involved in the two techniques. That entailing the use of a back flap is relatively safe, with only a 3 per cent chance of partial loss as a result of damage to the pedicle and the artery it carries, an occurrence necessitating eventual replacement of the dead tissue with a graft. The most frequent complication is the formation of a large blood clot in the back, but this can be avoided with the use of a drainage tube left in place for four to five days to drain off excess blood. Other complications likely to occur are those associated with a silicone prosthesis (see pp. 142–4).

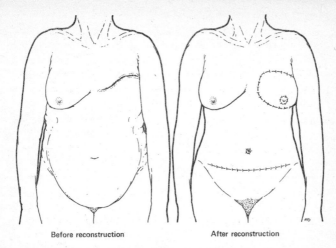

Before reconstruction   After reconstruction

Fig. 38 A new breast mound can also be created by means of a flap taken from the lower abdomen, a method which both has the added bonus of an abdomino-plasty and avoids the use of a silicone prosthesis, but which entails a greater risk of complications than that using a back flap. The nipple and areola are made with the aid of suitably pigmented skin grafts.

Scarring is of course inevitable, both in the donor area on the back and on the reconstructed breast.

The abdominal flap is used less frequently in Britain than the back flap, since the substantially greater, 20 to 30 per cent chance of partial tissue loss involves not only the skin itself but also the underlying fat, which is discharged as an oily yellow liquid for several weeks. Apart from the distress and inconvenience this causes the patient, it also means that the bulk of the reconstructed mound is gradually lost. Added to this is the fact that the removal of muscle from the abdomen via the abdominal flap leaves a weakness in the abdominal wall which can later lead to a hernia even if the remaining muscles have been reinforced. Nonetheless, this particular reconstructive technique is becoming increasingly popular in the USA, possibly because patients there are drawn by the allure of the built-in abdominoplasty, which unfortunately has its own complications as described in Chapter 16.

Whichever flap is used the sutures are removed after twelve days, but patients are advised to wait at least four weeks before returning to work or a full domestic routine. If the reconstructed breast does not completely match the other in size or shape, as can sometimes happen given the complexity of the technique, a compromise must be made and the healthy breast reduced if it is too large or tightened if it is too loose. This of course means further complications and scars, but minor adjustments can help to achieve the fundamental goal of providing a woman with a breast mound that is as similar as possible to the opposite breast, so that she can abandon her external prosthesis, display a balanced cleavage, and equally fill both cups of her bra or bikini. Of course she will deceive neither herself nor her partner in the privacy of her home, for the new breast will be dome- rather than cone-shaped and cannot possibly function like the original.

A nipple/areola complex can be created once the reconstructed breast has settled down, usually after three months, although few women who have undergone mastectomy and breast reconstruction are keen to go through yet another operation; many are quite happy to wear an adherent artificial nipple under their clothing instead.

The areola is made from a disc-shaped skin graft taken from the upper inner thigh, the nipple from a graft taken either from the nipple on the opposite breast, if there is enough to spare, or from the earlobe. The operation is quick and easy to perform, and is carried out under local or general anaesthesia with the patient as a day case. The only drawbacks are a scar in the donor area and fading of the new areola after a year.

If a woman thinking of breast reconstruction is disheartened by the description of the procedures and hazards involved and continues to have doubts after one or more consultations with the surgeon, she should certainly not go through with the operation, for unless wholly committed she is unlikely to be happy with the reconstructed breast, which will neither look exactly like the original nor function like it. Even so it must be said that a breast-shaped mound is very often preferable to an external prosthesis and a flat, scarred chest wall, and unquestionably invaluable to patients who find it difficult, if not impossible, to cope with the loss of their breast. More important, if women were more completely informed about the possibilities of reconstruction, those for whom the dread of mastectomy is greater than the fear of cancer itself would perhaps seek treatment sooner and thus possibly provide more favourable conditions for treatment.

[18]

Changing Sex

Many people, including some surgeons, doctors and nurses, find it impossible to accept the justification for a sex change, or that the few men and women who undergo the operation do so out of necessity rather than because they are disturbed, publicity-seeking freaks. It may be difficult to understand the motivation for such a dramatic metamorphosis, but if more were known about the phenomenon of transsexualism the cynics and sniggerers might come to sympathize with and even help these patients in their new role.

Transsexuals are anatomically normal men or women who have the physical features of one sex but feel that they belong to the other. Some resent their particular sexual characteristics so strongly that they are prepared to undergo actual surgery in order to acquire those of the opposite sex, wanting nothing more than to live and work in their new role and to be accepted in this by the general community. The overwhelming sense of entrapment felt by these individuals is sensitively expressed by Jan Morris in her book *Conundrum* (Coronet, 1975), where she describes how, in her original male form, both in boyhood and as an adult, she *knew* she was a woman and consequently felt herself ensnared in an alien body. In 1928 the phenomenon was described as aesthetic inversion, or eonism after the eighteenth-century French political adventurer Éon de Beaumont, otherwise known as the Chevalier d'Éon, who throughout much of his later life posed as a woman. As late as the early 1950s transsexualism was still lumped together with transvestism and homosexuality, but in the 1960s it became clear that, although there is some overlap, the three types of behaviour are very different.

A male transvestite (transvestism is very rare in females) derives pleasure from dressing as a woman, usually in private but occasionally in public. While some take a small further step and use hormones to increase the size of their breasts, they neither wish to live as women nor would they ever go so far as to have their genitalia removed. A homosexual, on the other hand, is sexually attracted to members of the same sex and sometimes adopts feminine or masculine mannerisms and postures traditionally associated with the opposite sex, with the aim of heightening the relationship with his or her partner. Both male and female homosexuals obtain sexual satisfaction through their own organs and would no more allow these to be surgically tampered with than they would have their heads cut off.

Although transsexuals may at some stage undergo a transient, usually experimental, period of homosexuality, as a rule, and until they commit themselves to change, the majority lead a normal, heterosexual life. Transvestism, on the other hand, becomes a permanent feature of their lives as they begin to establish their new identity, a feature that can neither be separated from their experience nor regarded as fetishism.

According to the classical criteria for establishing sexual status, a transsexual has the normal complement of male or female chromosomes, normal ovaries or testes, appropriate hormone levels, normal internal and external genitalia, and a body image to match, all adding up to either one or the other biological sex. Where the difference lies is in his or her psychosexual orientation, which is so at odds with the rest as to make him or her identify absolutely with the opposite gender. Thus an anatomical and biological male transsexual has such a strong sense of femininity that he will see himself as female, and vice versa.

Swedish figures indicate that the incidence of transsexualism is four times greater in females than in males, amounting to 1 in 30,000 for men and 1 in 120,000 for women. It is believed that there are more than 10,000 transsexuals living in Britain, although less than 1,000 have undergone surgery for transformation.

The true causes of transsexualism are unknown but there are two theories. The first proposes an abnormal hormonal environment influencing the child before birth so that a baby destined to be biologically male will develop behaviourally as a female. This theory has support from animal experiments in which monkeys were treated *in utero* with the opposite sex hormones and found, after birth, to behave in a transsexual fashion. However, this has not been substantiated in humans, and boys who, for reasons other than experimental, have received excessive oestrogen (female hormone) during the mother's pregnancy have briefly exhibited effeminate behaviour but experienced no gender crises as such.

The second theory, which although more convincing where male transsexuals are concerned remains unproven, holds that transsexualism arises when a boy is reared predominantly by a woman, his mother, who is herself anxious about role and gender and responds by reinforcing and overstressing her femininity, the father remaining a remote or absent figure throughout. The boy gradually asssumes female characteristics, both in fantasy and in reality, until he identifies wholly with the opposite gender. It is thought that the transfer of identity is complete by the third year, corresponding to the period in which language is developed.

Whatever the underlying cause, transsexualism makes its presence known in the first ten years of life with the child feeling that he or she is somehow different from others; dressing up may form part of this early phase. This is followed by actual and close identification with the opposite sex, which may be resisted in adult life with the individual trying to live in the gender that matches his or her physical sex and even marrying and having children. This role is not always maintained and symptoms relating to his or her intrinsic transsexualism may eventually attract the attention of a doctor, who may then set in motion the procedure for gender reassignment.*

Programme of Gender Reassignment

Gender identity once established is impossible to change, and attempts by psychiatrists to reverse adult transsexualism are not only useless but occasionally harmful. However, psychotherapy and medical treatment will help patients who, although they exhibit some or all of the symptoms, are not genuine transsexuals; these include psychotics deluded as to their sexual identity who may actually try to cut off their own sexual organs, sociopathic exhibitionists who look to a sex change as a means of obtaining personal notoriety through the media, and schizoid personalities who because they feel inadequate and overstressed in their present gender believe they can cope better in the other. Since gender reassignment is absolutely contra-indicated in all these cases, the psychiatrist must, to

---

* The term 'gender reassignment' is better than 'sex change'. The basic crisis is one of gender identity, and although a convincing transsexual physique may be created, the sex itself as determined genetically by the male or female chromosomes remains unchanged. Furthermore, in Britain, a birth certificate cannot be altered: in the eyes of the British law, once a male or female, always a male or female.

avoid disasters, assess patients very carefully and distinguish clearly between those who are genuinely motivated and those who are not.

To qualify for treatment, patients, as well as being suitably motivated, should be unmarried, twenty-one to fifty-five years old and physically fit. More important, they must understand two things: firstly, that the programme (if conducted by a reputable clinic) will take not less than three years to complete, will be irreversible, and will involve enormous social, professional and personal turmoil in the long transitional period; secondly, that, before being accepted for treatment, they will have to prove their suitability by living and working successfully in their new role (wearing the clothes of the opposite sex and undergoing appropriate hormone therapy) for at least a year and being entirely self-supporting during this time. This is the critical test and nine out of ten patients will either fail to qualify or have no further wish for surgery.

Like anyone undergoing cosmetic surgery, transsexual patients must not have unrealistic expectations. A solidly built man over six feet tall with size eight hands and size twelve feet will never pass easily as a woman, nor, even though the physical accoutrements of the original gender can be removed or disguised, will the surgically constructed organs of the new gender ever be particularly convincing, especially in the female transsexual. Patients must also accept that their transformation will be accompanied by serious risks and drawbacks, inevitable with such a major undertaking.

Given the complexity of the treatment, it is not surprising that the team caring for the patient is a large one, consisting of the psychiatrist, an endocrinologist (a doctor specializing in hormonal disorders), various surgeons, the patient's GP and a psychiatric social worker, and supported by counselling organizations, occupational therapists, patients who have already undergone gender reassignment, and sympathetic friends and relatives. The surgery itself is usually performed either by a urologist or a plastic surgeon, and since it is by far the least frequent of all cosmetic procedures will be more briefly outlined than the operations in previous chapters.

Male-to-Female Surgery

Although male transsexuals believe themselves to be female, they have great difficulty learning the correct gestures and mannerisms and, unless properly instructed, can acquire a grotesquely exaggerated and inappropriate manner. The first stage of the transformation is therefore spent teaching the patient with the help of other transsexuals how to develop a convincing female persona. Photographs and video tapes complement the lessons, and a tape of a transsexual interacting with other men and women in a social situation is invaluable in clearly pointing out to him all the subtle modifications necessary to make the transition. The adult male voice cannot be changed by hormone therapy or surgery but its timbre and pitch can be altered with the assistance of a speech therapist to give an attractive husky quality. The patient will find a tape recorder very useful for practising at home.

The second stage involves a course of hormone treatments and usually coincides with the one- to two-year trial period of living as a woman. The active female hormone used is oestrogen, which over a matter of eighteen months induces a redistribution of fat around the hips and thighs, increases the amount of breast tissue, reduces the size of the testes, improves the tone and texture of the skin, softens body and scalp hair and diminishes libido. Unwanted effects can include emotional instability, nausea, vomiting and dizziness. Unfortunately hormone therapy has no impact on facial hair and the only way to get rid of this is by electrolysis, which is tedious, time-consuming, uncomfortable and leaves tiny punctate scars.

If at the end of this stage the patient wishes to proceed with surgery and the management team judges him suitable, surgical gender reassignment can begin. The main goal is to construct a vulva and a vagina, and the surgeon starts by making a large pocket – the new vagina – between the rectum, the neck of the bladder and the urethra (the duct discharging urine from the bladder). The testes and penis are removed, the scrotal skin being retained to form the labia and the sheath of penile skin turned inside out to form the lining of the neo-vagina in conjunction with a split-skin graft. The end of the shortened urethra is then re-sited. After the tissues have settled, the new vagina must be regularly dilated with a tailor-made instrument to prevent it from contracting, even if it is being used in sexual intercourse. Narrowing of the vagina is in fact the commonest complication, followed by scarring, distortion and constriction of the relocated urethra. The space between the male rectum and urethra is obviously not intended to accommodate a vagina and is much smaller than in a woman, so that in making a pocket here there is a danger of piercing one or both of these structures, with disastrous and embarrassing consequences resolvable only by additional and somewhat extensive surgery. An alternative method of lining the vagina is to use a segment of bowel transferred from the pelvis; this entails a smaller risk of vaginal contraction but can cause excessive secretion of mucus.

Additional procedures such as facelift, eyelid reduction, breast augmentation and chin and nose reduction may be needed to provide the finishing touches (for details see appropriate chapters); the patient can also have the cartilages forming a prominent Adam's apple reduced.

Female-to-Male Surgery

The first stage of a female transsexual's transformation into a male entails a learning process similar to that already described for the male transsexual whereby the patient gradually acquires characteristics appropriate to her new role. This phase of the treatment is supplemented with bodybuilding exercises. Treatment with testosterone, a male hormone, in the second stage rapidly suppresses menstruation, increases body weight and encourages growth of body and facial hair, so that by the end of six months the patient may actually pass as a credible male.

If the patient is subsequently accepted for surgery, the first step will be to excise the breast tissues, using the same technique as that for gynaecomastia (enlargement of the male breasts), and to remove the ovaries and uterus. Construction of a penis is the next step, although not all patients in fact opt for this, particularly since a variety of prosthetic substitutes are available. If a full transformation is desired, however, the patient must undergo a lengthy and complex series of operations whose end result is a clumsy apparatus which functions solely as a conduit for urine. This method obviously has its drawbacks, but a surgical technique has recently been developed which allows a penis of approximately normal shape and size to be constructed and, moreover, to be erected by means of a solid silicone rod inserted prior to intercourse. A scrotum-like structure can also be provided by rearranging the labial tissues into a pouch and implanting two silicone prostheses as substitutes for testicles.

Transsexualism and the Law

The committed transsexual should apply for legal permission to change his or her name at an early stage, since only then can gender-specific documents such as the patient's driving licence, national insurance card and passport be adapted to match the new identity. If necessary, relevant medical evidence may be submitted in support of the application.

Although gender reassignment has many controversial aspects and is opposed on ethical grounds by many within the medical profession, an internationally recognized centre specializing in this form of treatment has demonstrated that the latter can be extremely beneficial in certain cases, and that 70 per cent of patients in fact show dramatic improvement in terms of social, psychological, economic and sexual function. Yet under British law the birth certificate cannot be amended and a transsexual who has undergone gender reassignment is still regarded by law as belonging to his or her original biological sex. This can lead to serious difficulties. For example, a marriage contract between a man and a male-to-female transsexual is considered null; a male transsexual undergoing his trial period as a woman may be seen as committing a breach of the peace in spite of the 'offence' being a medically acknowledged part of the treatment; a male-to-female transsexual cannot be given a state pension until the age of sixty-five while the female-to-male transsexual receives one at sixty; if sent to prison a transsexual may be forced to join prisoners of his or her original sex and possibly be deprived of essential hormone treatment.

The USA, Sweden and West Germany have recognized that properly supervised gender reassignment is a valid form of treatment and have passed legislation giving transsexuals the right to legal status in their new role. No such legislative change has so far been mooted within British law, although the question is under consideration in the European Court of Human Rights.

Appendix A:

Routes to Surgery in Britain

While self-advertising private cosmetic clinics offering clients a virtually instant service free of the need for referral are common in many countries, in Britain they are few and far between. The routes of referral in this country may seem unnecessarily and irritatingly complex, but they are there to protect patients' interests, safeguarding them as far as possible against the risks and complications of cosmetic surgery and against unscrupulous cosmetic surgeons. Any registered medical practitioner can put up his professional plate and practise in private as a cosmetic surgeon, regardless of background, previous experience or failure to acquire higher surgical qualifications; and professional bodies such as the General Medical Council responsible for maintaining and raising standards of medical care have no power to prevent him from operating on patients. Only if it is proved beyond doubt that there has been a serious breach of established ethical and professional standards is it in fact possible for such a doctor to be removed from the medical register and banned from further practice, and even then the ban applies only for a limited time, the doctor being quite at liberty to reapply for registration and resume work thereafter. Thus prospective patients must both be wary of putting themselves in the hands of the nearest and most accessible cosmetic surgeon and try if possible to follow those routes which have been carefully charted for them.

First of all they must consult the key figure, their general practitioner, who is the only person able to recommend a reputable surgeon and guide them safely through the system. If they have not already registered with a GP they must take steps to do so, since mistakes can happen if the system is bypassed – whether through embarrassment, shame, fear or impatience – and an appointment sought directly with a cosmetic surgeon. Although before the visit patients should have a clear idea as to their particular problem, they should, during the interview itself, avoid making immediate demands to see a cosmetic surgeon. While the GP cannot refuse a patient the right to seek specialist advice there are more tactful ways of making the request, and the patient is unwise to antagonize the person most likely to be involved in his care on discharge from hospital, as well as in other medical matters. The GP's answer will be based on what he knows of the character, medical history, domestic circumstances and family history of the patient, and if the pointers are not good he may well decide that cosmetic surgery is not the best form of treatment and that a second non-surgical opinion is needed in any case. However, if the request is reasonable, and after taking into account the patient's own preferences for a particular hospital or specialist, the GP will write to the cosmetic surgeon most appropriate for the job, giving not only the reasons for referral but also any background information relevant to the case. This letter is particularly important, since usually the consultant surgeon will refuse to see the patient without some kind of reference from the GP; even if a consultation does take place, the surgeon will not plan any treatment until he has communicated with him and received a satis-factory reply. This is not merely standard medical etiquette but a time-honoured, fail-safe mechanism, whose purpose is both to protect the patient from misunderstandings and mismanagement, and to provide continuity of care between medically qualified professionals working in the hospital environment and those working in the community at large.

Very occasionally patients will find themselves confronted with a general practitioner who is unsympathetic to their needs and who not only refuses to refer them to a cosmetic surgeon but also denies any other form of help. Such an attitude, which stems from prejudice, ignorance (cosmetic surgery is less frequently requested and performed in Britain than in other countries and is thus something of an unknown for a few doctors), or simply an unfavourable opinion based on one or two poor results, is fortunately quite rare, but even if they experience it patients should not be deterred, for they are completely entitled to a second opinion. In a group practice, this can often be obtained from another partner, who may well be both better informed and more sympathetic.

Once the appointment has been made and the patient finally reaches the surgeon's consulting room, he must once again explain the nature of the problem, answer relevant questions and undergo medical tests. If the surgeon, having listened to and examined the patient and studied both the GP's letter and any hospital records relating to previous admissions or treatment, concludes that the proposed surgical treatment is both safe and justifiable, he will explain the pros and cons outlined in the Surgical Gazetteer and, with the patient's consent, make arrangements for the operation. The final decision does not have to be made instantly and if, following the interview, the patient has second thoughts about undergoing surgery, he can ask for time to ponder further and to discuss the matter with friends and relatives. On the other hand, if some aspect of the patient's health, attitude or medical history leads to reservations on the surgeon's part as to the advisability of proceeding further, he will in all likelihood deem it proper to engage the help of a specialist colleague. Thus a diabetic will be referred to a physician, an individual suffering from heart disease or high blood pressure to a cardiologist, and a patient with what seem to be underlying neurotic or psychotic symptoms to a psychiatrist. The specialist's report will give the surgeon a better picture of the patient's condition and enable him to make the right decision.

If surgery is contra-indicated, the consultant will explain the reasons. The patient is not, however, obliged to accept these, and has every right to seek referral elsewhere for a second opinion. This can be arranged either by the first surgeon or by the patient's GP. If the second surgeon takes the same view, the patient will be well advised to abandon the idea of surgery, however distressing this may be. The point cannot be made too frequently firstly that cosmetic surgery is neither life-saving nor absolutely essential, and that risks which can be taken in an emergency cannot reasonably be taken here; and secondly that patients who continue to shop around having twice been refused and who eventually find someone somewhere – as they undoubtedly will – who agrees to operate, will quite possibly end up not only paying a large sum they can ill afford but also bitterly regretting the whole venture.

Whether an operation is carried out through the National Health Service or in the private sector, both the pattern of referral and the quality of surgery and in-patient care are very similar. But there are also important differences, especially for the patient wanting cosmetic surgery. Although the NHS was introduced in 1948 to provide comprehensive medical care to all British citizens regardless of their financial means, this idealistic dream has proved difficult to realize in the 1980s. Certainly in emergencies or where there is an obvious need for treatment the NHS with its high standard of care remains one of the best medical systems in the world, but where non-urgent treatment is concerned the picture is somewhat different. Indeed, patients with what is regarded as a low-priority illness can find themselves waiting a long time between seeing their GP and seeing the specialist and, if surgery is planned, a very long time indeed between the interview and admission, whose date will inevitably have been set to fit in with the hospital schedule rather than their own. They will eventually be treated, but the wait may well be lengthy, unpredictable and extremely frustrating.

Regardless of how strongly patients may feel that they deserve cosmetic surgery, this form of treatment cannot possibly constitute a priority in the context of other, more urgent forms within the NHS. It is also very clear that other patients subscribing through taxes to the NHS, and doctors working within it, resent the fact that they may be underwriting a facelift or an eyelid reduction and that those undergoing such an operation are obstructing the admission of others who are perhaps more deserving of treatment. Although under the National Health Act of 1946 there is nothing to prevent anyone from having cosmetic surgery under the NHS, it has to be understood that all patients desiring this kind of treatment must inevitably take their turn in a very long queue which, depending on the district in which they live, may leave them waiting several months and even many years for admission to hospital.

Not surprisingly, then, a large number of patients look to the private sector for help, since here they can have exactly the operation they want when they want it, and also enjoy a substantial measure of privacy and luxury at the same time. However, there are potential hazards in this system, and particularly in the selection of the cosmetic surgeon.

The majority of surgeons working in private practice are also consultants in the National Health Service, a position achieved after lengthy training in a competitive, pyramidal system from which they emerge as fully qualified and accredited specialists, but there are also those who work exclusively in the private sector. While a few of these will once have been NHS consultants, most are not accredited by the Royal College of Surgeons in any speciality. To add to the confusion, no training system in surgery is foolproof, and there is no guarantee that a fully accredited surgeon with a string of higher qualifications will be a faultless exponent of the trade. Likewise there is no reason why a surgeon who has failed to stay the full course of recognized training and who has chosen at an early stage to work entirely in the private sector should not, by dint of experience, eventually become very able. In order to avoid mistakes, patients should be careful when selecting a private surgeon to rely as fully as possible on their GP and to follow the recommendations of others who have undergone similar treatment.

Another unavoidable disadvantage of private cosmetic surgery is that it is expensive and – with the possible exception of breast reconstruction after mastectomy and revision of unacceptable scars resulting from accidents, burns or previous surgery; skin tumours suspected or known to be malignant; birthmarks; prominent ears in children; jaw and nose deformities due to accidental injury; birth defects; extremes of developmental disproportion and breast asymmetry – unlikely to be covered by any health-insurance policy.* Unfortunately, fees vary so enormously from one procedure, surgeon and region to another that it is quite outside the scope of this book to give a probable cost for any one cosmetic operation, and it is up to the patient himself to obtain a written estimate of the total cost, including surgeon's, assistant's and anaesthetist's fees and the cost of hospitalization and follow-up appointments, before embarking on treatment. Only thus can later distress and unpleasantness be avoided.

---

* To ascertain if a particular operation is covered by his policy, the patient should contact the relevant insurance company; if the answer is in the affirmative, written confirmation should be obtained and kept for future reference.

Appendix B:

Consent, Complaint and Redress

There are no perfect arrangements for health care in any part of the world, and regardless of the political system of a country, the availability and wealth of its resources and the efficiency of its administration, agreed standards are not always maintained, which means that mistakes can happen. The National Health Service is aware of the possibility of error and has built into its structure a mechanism not only for answering and investigating patients' complaints but also for acting on them, should they be well founded, in order to reduce the chances of the fault recurring. Doctors and surgeons are equally aware of their fallibility and subscribe to medical defence organizations to represent them in the event of a patient taking legal action and to pay or contribute to any damages awarded against them.

Health authorities in England in fact receive remarkably few complaints, and of the sixteen million or so NHS patients treated per year only about fifteen thousand (representing less than 0.1 per cent) actually initiate a formal, and in most cases minor, complaint. This number could be further reduced if the implications and common hazards of a particular treatment were clearly understood by every patient. Unfortunately, not all surgeons take care to explain an operation and its risks in comprehensible terms, and patients often fail either to grasp their meaning or to air their worries and queries, instead taking everything, including a perfect result, for granted. This obviously leads to problems: surgeons engaged in cosmetic surgery are notoriously vulnerable to complaints and litigation, not necessarily because of any mistakes but more often because inadequately informed patients have unrealistic expectations which cannot be fulfilled, and seek a second opinion or even legal advice without giving the original surgeon a chance to help.

Proper communication between the surgeon and patient is crucial from first to last if a mutually satisfactory result is to be achieved, and failure to reach an understanding can lead to nothing but resentment and hostility on either side. One of the purposes of this book has been to show what can realistically be expected of cosmetic surgery; another must be to appeal to patients to find out from the surgeon exactly what they are letting themselves in for and to discuss any subsequent misgivings or worries fully before signing the consent form.

Consent to Treatment

Consent is essential for surgical treatment. To exercise effectively this fundamental right to self-determination, the patient must be given enough information about the proposed treatment to be able to make a rational and reasoned choice and to deny consent if need be. How much detail the surgeon gives of the treatment and its risks depends on several things, including the patient's understanding and the likelihood of such information causing further harm to his health. It may not be necessary, for example, to describe complications which occur only rarely or unlikely side-effects which a reasonable patient would not consider significant, and the explanation must achieve a realistic balance between the risks of the treatment and the possible consequences of its withholding. In cosmetic surgery the scales are obviously tipped decisively in the former direction, and the surgeon is therefore obliged to give more details of the drawbacks of treatment than would be the case, for example, with a patient about to have part of the lungs removed for cancer.

If a surgeon carries out an operation for which consent has not been given he is liable both to be prosecuted for assault under the criminal law and to be sued for damages, such an operation constituting trespass to the person. In emergencies, however, exceptions can be made and surrogate consent obtained from the patient's next-of-kin; if no one can be found to give this, the surgeon may be free to assume implied consent and to proceed with treatment. Implied consent applies, for example, in the case of an unconscious person brought to a casualty department by ambulance and suffering from multiple injuries sustained in a car accident, including life-threatening trauma such as a ruptured liver or brain damage. The character and severity of the injuries and the urgency of admission to hospital are such that the necessity for treatment is assumed and consent immediately taken for granted. The surgeon can then act to the benefit of the patient without fear of prosecution. Implied consent does not apply to patients about to undergo cosmetic surgery, and in their case verbal or written, i.e., expressed, consent needs to be obtained.

Oral consent can be given by the patient for the removal of, for instance, a skin lesion such as a small mole, i.e., when the procedure is a minor one and carried out under local anaesthesia with the patient conscious and fully aware of his surroundings. However, should the mole, on examination by a pathologist, prove to be a malignant tumour requiring more extensive surgery under general anaesthesia with all its added risks, written consent must be obtained. In fact the medical defence union advises its members: 'It should be the invariable practice to obtain the patient's written consent to any operation which requires a general anaes- thetic or to any procedure which involves a special risk.' Evidencing consent by signature is a simple matter. A standard form is used by all hospitals in the United Kingdom and is signed by the patient in the presence of the doctor. If there is anything on the form with which the patient does not agree he can simply modify the wording before sign- ing.

From the above it is clear that there are a number of vague terms and definitions which raise important legal questions. Exactly how much information is a doctor required to give? When can a patient be judged 'informed' and capable of making a 'rational' decision? Lawyers in the USA quickly recognized these weaknesses and, realizing that charges of 'assault and battery' and 'failure to warn' would in many cases be easier to substantiate than surgical incompetence or negligence, began to exploit the loopholes to the benefit of clients who had suffered complications during surgical treatment. Vitiating the patient's consent and thus the legality of the treatment by bringing doubt to bear on the completeness of the information supplied by the surgeon, they often succeeded in rendering him liable to damages for assault and battery. The process of interpreting informed consent became so labyrinthine and judicial policy began to turn so much in favour of the patient that, to protect themselves against malpractice suits and to avoid creating loopholes, surgeons had no choice but to list in considerable detail the potential dangers of any operation, whilst conducting exhaustive medical investigations that were of more use to their attorney in the event of litigation than to the patient himself. The situation was further complicated by the fact that American lawyers are paid contingency fees amounting to a certain percentage of the final settlement, which is an incentive to make outrageous financial demands for compensation. As a result, malpractice insurance premiums paid annually by surgeons rocketed to such ridiculous levels (in some states surgeons in more vulnerable fields such as orthopaedic and plastic surgery continue to pay up to a hundred thousand dollars a year) that in certain cases they even exceeded the surgeon's yearly income. The farcical aspects of this situation were highlighted by car stickers appealing to parents, 'Send your children to medical school and feed a lawyer.'

Informed consent in the USA became 'ill-informed consent' as the growing practice of defensive medicine, encouraged by surgeons' fear of prosecution, by their awareness of the increasing abuse of the system at the hands of unscrupulous individuals, and by their desire to cover all eventualities, began to work against patients' well-being, with surgeons expounding far more the dangers than the benefits of treatment, thereby causing patients unnecessary anxiety and distress and putting paid to any possibility of rational decision-making or informed consent.

The interpretation of informed consent has since been modified in the USA, but even in its present form it would be unacceptable in Britain, where contingency fees are unethical and illegal and where judicial policy is quite different. Although there are admitted weaknesses in the definition of informed consent in Britain it is to be hoped that whatever changes may be made will not adversely influence the way surgeons currently investigate and treat their patients.

Complaint and Redress

Having accepted that there is no Utopian system of health care and that mistakes can happen, one must also accept that the patient, as a consumer, has every right to complain if some aspect of his care has been deficient or if unnecessary suffering has followed treatment. Unfortunately, patients tend to be deterred from initiating a complaint both by reports of the hostile closing of ranks by medical and administrative staff, which does nothing to help their confidence, and by a lack of information as to the manner for proceeding. In fact very clear instructions for reporting and handling complaints are issued to hospitals by the Department of Health and Social Security with the aim not only of providing a speedy solution but also of reducing the likelihood of any such complaint recurring. After all, the NHS is there to benefit patients as well as the people working within it, and it is only fair that the consumer should be allowed to air any misgivings and to help improve the standard of care for future patients.*

Most complaints are minor, relating to disenchantment with food, bureaucracy or the hospital routine, and can usually be resolved directly by approaching the relevant staff and requesting them to put matters right. Should the patient be dissatisfied with this, however, he can submit a formal complaint either verbally or in writing to the relevant member of the hospital administration, who has instructions 'to investigate the problem as thoroughly, fairly and quickly as circumstances permit and to keep the complainant and any persons complained about fully and promptly informed of reasons for unavoidable delay in resolving the issue'. If there is still no satisfactory outcome the patient may then complain to the Health Service Commissioner (also known as the NHS ombudsman), who has a parliamentary duty to investigate any complaint providing that it has already been made to the local district health authority, that it is made in writing and within one year of the incident, and that it is not being taken to a tribunal or law court. While the commissioner cannot investigate complaints bearing on a doctor's clinical judgement, surgical competence or the effects of treatment, and can never adjudicate on compensation, which is a matter for the courts, he is bound by law to answer any relating to maladministration and defects in the service such as poor ward or hospital conditions or failure to provide a service at all, for instance in an out-patients' or accident department. If a patient is uncertain whether a complaint can be taken up by the commissioner, he can either write to him for advice or ask for help from the Community Health Council or the Citizens' Advice Bureau. 95 per cent of all formal complaints can in fact be dealt with locally and only about 700 actually reach the commissioner in any year. Of these roughly one third are upheld, when a recommendation is made to the health authority to apologize to the patient, to change or improve a particular hospital procedure, or to reimburse the patient in the event of loss or damage to property.

If a patient has any queries or doubts about the treatment itself, by far the best solution is to broach the subject directly with the surgeon or the nursing and surgical staff involved. Most problems in this area are rooted simply in a failure to communicate, whether on one or both sides, so that uninhibited discussion of misgivings will usually be enough to resolve any

* Anyone who wishes to know more about the health service should read *Patients' Rights*, published in 1983 by the National Consumer Council, and *A Patient's Guide to the National Health Service*, published also in 1983 by the Consumers' Association and Hodder & Stoughton.

difficulty. However, if the surgeon does not manage to give a satisfactory answer, the patient can write to the Regional Medical Officer (RMO), who will investigate the circumstances before making a decision and possibly ask the consultant to try once more to clarify matters. Should even this advice be unhelpful and the patient feel strongly enough to take legal action, he can initiate a third stage called an independent professional review and thus obtain what amounts to a second opinion. In this case the RMO arranges for two independent consultants in the relevant speciality to assess the case and meet the aggrieved party as well as any relative or friend who might also wish to attend. The original consultant need not be present but may be invited to appear at some stage in the proceedings. The two consultants then send a confidential report to the RMO, who writes back to the patient, with a copy to the consultant, explaining what decision has been reached and what action, if any, will be taken.

While the procedure for lodging a complaint is much the same in England, Wales, Scotland and Northern Ireland, the established channels are open only to NHS patients and to private patients using pay beds in an NHS hospital, no formal routes existing in the private sector. What is perhaps more significant is that no complaints procedure whatsoever leads to financial compensation, and if patients feel that they have suffered needlessly during or following treatment and deserve some form of recompense, their only course of action may be to institute legal proceedings. Prior to this step, of course, they should consult a solicitor or an organization offering help to individuals who believe they have reasonable grounds for proving medical negligence (either Action for the Victims of Medical Accidents or the National Association of Compensation Claimants).

Faults and flaws obviously do exist in the present complaints procedure and patients often feel unjustly treated. For this reason the DHSS is keen that a new and more open system should be implemented, and in a press release following a meeting of the forum of health-care professions in January 1983, Mr Kenneth Clark, the Minister of Health, stated: 'With these initiatives, I hope to see the National Health Service shed some of its very largely unfair reputation for closing up like a clam at the first mention of complaint, fault or possible litigation. I do not believe that a policy of greater openness will encourage litigation. But I do believe that a defensive attitude could well stimulate a litiginous one. When things go wrong, there are many alternative avenues apart from litigation, and I am convinced that it is in the interests of us all to explore them more openly and honestly.'